Devizes Union

from Workhouse to Hospital

1836 - 1990

BARBARA FULLER

First published in the United Kingdom in 2016 for the Author, Barbara Fuller, by The Hobnob Press, 30c Deverill Road Trading Estate, Sutton Veny, Warminster BA12 7BZ www.hobnobpress.co.uk

British Library Cataloguing in Publication Data
A catalogue record for this book is available from the British Library

ISBN 978-1-906978-40-2

Typeset in Adobe Garamond Pro 11/14 pt. Typesetting and origination by John Chandler.

Printed by Lightning Source

Contents

Acknowledgements		5
Foreword		7
1	The Setting up of the Devizes Union	11
2	Children – Workhouse Inmates	26
3	Children – Boarded-Out	35
4	Guardians, Committees and Staff	57
5	Physical and Mental Health and Causes of Death both in the House and those receiving Out-Relief	73
6	Settlements and Removals	90
7	Out-Relief	101
8	Problems	110
9	Vagrants	129
10	Wartime and Aftermath	144
11	St James Hospital	151
12	Incidentals	166
13	Reminiscences	182
14	Bertie Bushnell	194
	Bibliography	199
	Index of Surnames	200

Acknowledgements

The author would like to thank the following for their help and advice:

Cy and Scindia Cutler
Una Davies
Lyn Dyson
Dorothy Fox
Andy Geddes
John Hawkins
Lorna Haycock
John Hurley
The late Colin Kearley (photographs)
Jerry King
Ordnance Survey
Jean Philpott
Eileen Reeves
Miriam Smith
Bill Underwood
John Willett
Wiltshire Archeological & Natural History Society (Library)
Wiltshire Family History Society
Wiltshire & Swindon History Centre Staff

Contributors to 1986 booklet, *Changed Times* – Peggy Dyke, Jane King, Violet Murray, George Waistell.

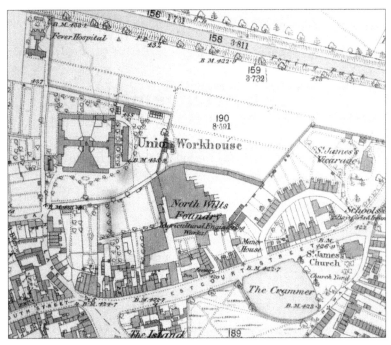

Plans showing the buildings in the 1880s (Ordnance survey) and the 1960s (Wessex Regional Health Authority)

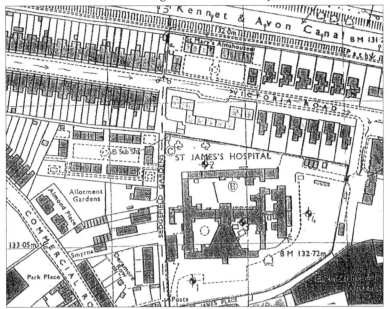

Foreword

In 1986 I was asked to produce a booklet for some celebrations to be held to mark the 150th anniversary of the building which had originally been Devizes Union Workhouse up to its hospital status. This led to the printing of *Changed Times*, the title taken from the comments of a nurse who was able to tell me about his experiences. I have never lost my interest in the history of the change from Workhouse to hospital, the lives of the people who had to take advantage of the 'hospitality' in the Workhouse, also those who qualified for out-relief, up to the humane hospital regime when it became a geriatric hospital, although even at this later date many of the older residents of the town still thought of its past history as the workhouse with a feeling of horror.

I also have other connections with the site as I worked for a short time at St James Hospital in 1965 and was involved with the building and management of St James surgery which now occupies part of the site.

Each chapter starts with a brief introduction followed by actual entries from the Minute Books. Hopefully this will bring some of the people to life and not just as statistics caught in the system.

The Minute books of the Board of Guardians give quite an insight into what life might have been like for those unfortunates who needed help. Whilst the books give great insight into the attitudes of the Guardians towards the Workhouse inmates (sometimes harsh, sometimes enlightened) even they were constrained by the rules and regulations imposed by the Government and they often had to consult the Poor Law Commissioner for advice or permission. The Minute books also give a one-sided idea of what was going on although, just occasionally, the voice of a pauper appears when they make a complaint against conditions or one of the staff – often dismissed but occasionally leading to some changes in procedures.

A new Poor Law was enacted by Parliament in 1834 due to the fact that poor relief was becoming increasingly expensive. A solution was sought to provide a uniform system under a central authority with the parish still responsible to pay the poor rates. Then, as today, there was the fear that this was encouraging people to take advantage and that some were not the 'deserving' poor, and also by allowing parish relief employers could keep wages artificially low. The Poor Law Commissioners also disliked public benefactors as they 'disrupted discipline'.

The 1834 Act meant that parishes were lumped together into Unions with a Board of Guardians who had the duty to be in overall charge. They were to be elected by the ratepayers. The Devizes Union consisted of 28 parishes.

Everyone who applied for relief was to be assessed by a Relieving Officer who would decide if they were eligible after applying the workhouse test. The able bodied were only to get relief if they were admitted to the workhouse. Conditions in the house were to be harder than those for the common labouring family, known at the time as 'less eligibility'. In the 'Rules & Regulations' it stated that legally, any man who accepted relief from the poor rate became a pauper and lost his status as a citizen which meant he could not vote. However some outdoor relief continued for the old, infirm, sick, and widows with small children – they were the 'deserving' poor.

Entry to the House was meant to be dreaded and feared by the poor and it worked, at least initially. The 1834 Poor Law Act dramatically changed previous methods of Poor Relief and every Union was compelled to provide a Workhouse. Help was to be available inside the house and no more out-relief to be given to the able-bodied. Some parishes did not stick to the book and out-relief was still given, especially in the north where there was great opposition to the changes. The 1834 report gave the ultimatum that all relief whatever to able-bodied persons or their families otherwise than in a well-regulated workhouse (that is to say in places where they may be set to work according to the spirit and intention of the Act) would be declared unlawful. The aim of the system was that it should be a self-acting test which would not abolish relief but would ensure that only the truly destitute and helpless would receive it.

Seventeen union workhouses were set up in Wiltshire to comply with the 1834 Poor Law Act. These were Alderbury, Amesbury, Bradford-on-Avon, Calne, Chippenham, Cricklade and Wootton Bassett, Devizes, Highworth and Swindon, Malmesbury, Marlborough, Melksham, Mere, Pewsey, Tisbury, Warminster, Westbury and Whorwellsdown and Wilton.

A full list of the dates of the Devizes Union Minute Books can be seen at the Wiltshire & Swindon History Centre and they cover 1835 to 1930 with only four years missing (1846-1849), also the Minutes of the Boarding-Out Committee 1910-1927.

What follows is but a small example of what can be found in these Minute books plus some items from local newspapers, correspondence held at the National Archives, Kew, and personal reminiscences.

Barbara Fuller

MONEY WANTED,

On good Security, under the authority of an Act of Parliament.

THE GUARDIANS of the POOR of the DE-VIZES UNION are desirous of borrowing the sum of Five Thousand Six Hundred and Fifty Pounds, for which Security will be given, with the approbation of the Poor Law Commissioners, by charge on the Poor Rates of the Parishes of the Union, bearing interest at 4 per Cent.

This Sum must be repaid in the proportions, and at the times undermentioned ; and the Securities will therefore be made payable at such respective times, viz.:—

20th March, 1839	£350	20th March, 1850	£350
1840	350	1851	350
1841	350	1852	350
1842	350	1853	350
1843	350	1854	350
1844	350	1855	350
1847	350	1856	400
1848	350		
1849	350		£5650

The Money will be required on the 20th March next, from which time Interest will be paid Quarterly.

The Securities will be transferable without Stamp Duty.

Persons willing to advance all, or any part of the Money required, are requested to inform the Guardians thereof by letter (free of postage), mentioning the particular sums they are willing to advance (with reference to the times of repayment), to be left on or before the 11th December next, at the Clerk's Office, where all necessary information will be given.

By Order of the Board of Guardians,

W. E. TUGWELL, Clerk.

Devizes, 14th Nov., 1837.

Advert placed in the Devizes Gazette

1

The Setting up of the Devizes Union

On 7 November 1835, following the requirements of the 1834 Poor Law Amendment Act, the Guardians for the different parishes were elected (36 in all plus 6 ex-officio) and T.H.S.B.Estcourt was chosen to be Chairman of the Board of Guardians. Mr Edmund Tugwell was to be Clerk at a salary of £80 p.a. The occupations of the other elected Guardians were given as brewer, gentleman, cartwright, coal merchant, tinman, but the largest number were farmers. An Auditor and Treasurer were also appointed.

In March 1836 an order was sent by the Poor Law Commission directing that an advertisement be placed in the Devizes Gazette for the election of Guardians on 31 March and that notices should be printed and sent out to parish officers for posting on doors of churches and anywhere else parochial notices were usually displayed. Forms for the election were to be supplied at the expense of the Union. T.Estcourt was re-elected as Chairman and at the same time two other Committees were appointed – a Visiting Committee and a Building Committee. In October 1837 Estcourt sent a letter to his fellow Guardians stating his intention to resign from the Board as his Parliamentary and other duties prevented him from attending the meetings of the Guardians as frequently as he wished but his offer to resign was not accepted. His name is rarely mentioned again in the Minutes so presumably his decision to resign did not change, his Parliamentary duties taking precedence (he was M.P. for Devizes from 1835 until 1844).

After the election, meeting days and times were set and were to be held in the offices of Messrs Salmon, Tugwell and Meek. The Poor

Law Commissioner, Colonel A'Court, attended and gave averages for the taxation of each parish.

Devizes Union was split into 5 districts. The Relieving Officers with their yearly salaries are listed below.

District 1

Devizes St John, Devizes St James, Devizes St Mary (population 6327). Relieving Officer John Withers £80

District 2

Chittoe Tything, Bromham, Rowde, Poulshot (population 3140). Relieving Officer James Taylor £75

District 3

Bishops Cannings, All Cannings, Allington, Stanton St Bernard, Alton Barnes, Etchilhampton, Beechingstoke (population 3090). Relieving Officer Ed.Sloper £75

District 4

Potterne, Marston, Worton, West Lavington, Great Cheverell, Little Cheverell, Erlestoke (population 4224). Relieving Officer John Glass £80

District 5

Patney, Marden, Chirton, Urchfont, Market Lavington, Easterton, Stert Tything (population 3857). Relieving Officer Abraham Gray £90.

At this time Poor House accommodation was mainly in small properties with none large enough or suitable for a Union House. A committee was appointed to look at a possible scite (sic) for a Union Workhouse to accommodate 300-400. The small committee who were to investigate possible sites were Messrs. Salmon, Brown, Box and Smith. However, a temporary workhouse was needed until a site had been purchased, plans prepared and an architect and builder employed. A suitable building was found in New Park Street, Devizes, which had formerly been Anstie's Clothing Factory. The Board were offered the building for one year at a rent of £120. (This was the same building which in 1796 had been used as a House of Industry to employ the poor, with any proceeds to be used to provide food, beer and firing)

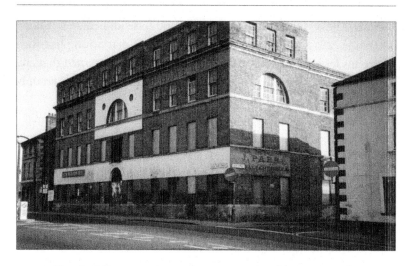

New Park Street premises used as temporary workhouse – now flats

Possible sites for the new building were investigated at Pans Lane (adjoining the Poor House called the Pest House), Back Lane (leading from Devizes Green to the canal wharf) plus other sites and including the London Turnpike Road and adjoining Gallows Lane. The Board decided on some ground belonging to the Trustees for the infant children of Thomas Burton and in 1836 received permission from the Poor Law Commission to go ahead and buy the site.

The Board had accepted the tender for one year's rent for the New Park Street building and on 28 December 1835 Mr William Cozens and Ann his wife were appointed as Master and Matron. They were warned not the think of themselves as tenants of the workhouse but merely to reside there at the discretion of the Board. They were directed to take their household furniture for their own private use into the Work House and that their salary would commence from 1 January. The Cozens were also ordered not to take in any pauper without an Order, and if they left a new Order was required for re-admission. No other staff appointments were made except for a porter. It was taken for granted that the paupers themselves would carry out any tasks required in relation to cleaning, laundry, kitchen work and nursing. An advert was duly put into the Devizes Gazette and John Strong, a labourer of Rowde, was appointed at £13 p.a. plus board and lodging – he was ordered to go to the Workhouse immediately. On 26 December 1837 it was reported in the Minutes that Strong had died of typhus fever. The Medical Officer did not seem concerned that any action needed to be taken regarding paupers in the house and certainly no other cases were reported in the minutes.

Early in January 1836 the parishes had been ordered to make lists of paupers, bastards, friendless children and any others considered to be suitable candidates for admission and it was planned initially to receive 50 paupers. On the 23 January it is noted that there were 5 men, 14 women, 7 girls and 4 boys in the House and that 3 men, 4 women, 1 boy and 2 girls had been discharged. By 1 February there were 33 paupers in the House but a week later numbers had risen to 64. By week 13 there were 90 inmates.

On 21 March 1836 the tender from John Goring and Benoni White for building the new Workhouse according to Mr Wilkinson's plan, but in brick not stone for £4,816, was accepted. The building work was to be completed by 20 October with a forfeit of £30 per week for over-running that date. The Clerk was to prepare the contract and explain it to the builders who agreed to supply labour. Another job was to apply to Parliament for relief of duty on bricks and materials for the Workhouse building.

In April the architect, Mr Wilkinson, had reported that the building work was proceeding and he was ordered by the Board to appoint a competent Clerk of Works immediately. However, this did not seem to go very well as William Schooler, Clerk of Works, was dismissed in mid- June as he had not attended his work for several days.

The contractors had asked about drains and it was decided that the architect's advice should be sought. In the meantime permission to use the sewers under terms of the Devizes Improvement Act had to be obtained. In answer to the query about drains the architect said that he had examined the levels on the site and that they could not be connected with the town sewers. Cesspools, according to specification, were then ordered. By going through a neighbours land they would be able to lay a waste water drain but this would cost them money in compensation. By early August application was made to the feoffees (trustees) of St Mary's for permission to lay a waste water drain from the new House through part of their land. The next month Mr Truman, through whose garden the new drain would run, had asked that either the soil should not be disturbed till his crop of potatoes was harvested or that the crop should be purchased. The Board decided to buy the potato crop for £3 as construction of the drains was urgent. Another neighbour, Robert Lavington, asked for compensation of £12 for the breaking down of his boundary fence in order to carry the sewer through. In February 1837 the Board had agreed to pay him £9 compensation and a dry well and cess pit were to be made to prevent further damage to the property. One member of the Board accused the architect of want of proper attention.

RULES AND REGULATIONS FOR RELIEF

Application was to be made to the relieving officer of the appropriate district. On admission – examination by the Medical Officer and his decision made if for sick ward or other according to class assigned.

Class 1 – Infirm through age or other causes.
Class 2 – Able-bodied above 15 years of age (men and youths).
Class 3 – Boys above 7 and under 15 years of age.
Class 4 – Women through age or other cause.
Class 5 – Able-bodied above 15 years of age (women and girls).
Class 6 – Girls above 7 and under 15 years of age.
Class 7 – Under 7's.

6 January 1835 – Mr Spackman of Bradford Union offered to supply clothing for men, women and children. He made up clothing for 10 men, 20 women and 20 children (10 boys and 10 girls) and was paid £197.14.0 for the work. The 'uniform' was to be worn at all times, including outside the Workhouse. A few days later a letter from an emigration officer at Manchester laid down the rule that no identifying mark should be put on Workhouse clothing without good reason. At another meeting in February 1836 more tenders were received by the Committee and providers of clothing were chosen. By March 1836

the Guardians decided that all Workhouse clothing should be marked with a proper marking instrument.

In order to get admitted to the House or receive out-relief the applicant would first have to get an Order from the Relieving Officer which the Guardians had the power to grant or refuse. If the family would only accept out-relief and refused admission to the house then they would get no help if, after decision of the Medical Officer, they were considered to be able-bodied.

ON ADMISSION

Before leaving the reception area the inmate was to be washed and their clothes removed and replaced with work-house clothing (their own clothes to be handed back when leaving unless they were inmates for a long period). However there was to be no mark degrading to the pauper in the clothes except something to establish it as the property of the Workhouse. The pauper was also to be thoroughly searched and any item prohibited by Act of Parliament removed. This included razors, knives and alcohol.

The Medical Officer would examine each person and if thought to be medically fit would decide their 'class' and ability to work. The sick would go to the infirmary and the pregnant to a lying-in ward. Unmarried mothers were the second largest group after the old. Up to at least the 1860s the lying-in wards were extremely primitive – it was not considered necessary to offer comforts as the unmarried inmates were there 'in consequence of their own sin'.

Men, their wives and children were separated – this was to be entire between the sexes with different parts of the House for eating, sleeping and living although infants could stay with their mothers until of school age. The inmates were told they could not leave except permanently, but this rule was often ignored and some paupers would return somewhat the worse for wear having somehow managed to get some money together which they had used to visit a local hostelry.

Once an inmate, the pauper was subjected to various rules, mainly pertaining to their behaviour. They were prohibited from making noise, using profane language, committing assault, pretending sickness, gambling, disobeying a lawful order made by an officer of the workhouse, climbing over the wall and refusal to wash. More serious offences included repeated disorderly behaviour, insulting the Master or Matron or the Guardians, disobeying a repeated order of the Master or Matron, fighting, damage to Guardians' property, spoiling provisions, getting drunk. If the case was serious enough referral to a Justice of the Peace would be made.

Shaving took place just once a week the same as bathing and there was no privacy as a member of staff had to be present in the bathroom.

Every morning the paupers would be woken by a bell and there would be a roll-call and prayers before breakfast. From Monday to Saturday the able-bodied would go to their allotted work with a one hour break for dinner followed by more prayers read by the Master then back to work, a ten hour day. Discipline and tedium was the aim

THE BUILDING

1836

In January the elected Board of Guardians had asked permission and received authority from the Commission to buy a piece of land on which to build a workhouse. After conferring with Col. A'Court, the Board of Guardians was directed to provide a statement of accounts after purchasing the land. Mr Thomas James Head, a local chemist of Devizes, loaned £1,000 at 4% interest to pay for this. On 18 January the Clerk was ordered to proceed with the purchase and arrange for the £1,000 security to be signed and sealed for when the conveyance was ready (cost of the land was £700). Seven architect's plans were received. Mr Wilkinson's was preferred and sent to the Poor Law Commission for approval.

In February the amount of money needed to be borrowed was £5,650. The Minutes list how this was to be repaid over 20 years at 4% interest and an advert was put into the papers seeking investors headlined 'Money Wanted'. On 26 March the Board paid out one quarter's interest which was due to Mr Finch, Mr Harding and Mr Box.

On 4 October Messrs Young and White, the contractors, delivered in W.Wilkinson's certificate of their being entitled to the further sum of £1,000 for building the new Workhouse. The Board, not having any funds requested Mr Tugwell to lend them the sum of £1,000 at 5% interest, which he had consented to do. On the 11 October it was noted that no permanent loan was to be taken out as Mr Tugwell had already loaned £2,750 and at the beginning of November he loaned another £1,250. The investors were later listed as John French of London, William Harding, Rowde Farm, Thomas Waldren of Eastridge, Thomas Waldron, Upper Lambourne, Berks and Lovegrove Waldron of Eastridge, Ramsbury. The totals were short of requirements by £700 but a further amount of £400 at 4% interest was loaned by Mr Thomas James Head.

By 21 November the builders had not finished and 142 paupers were still in the temporary Workhouse. The contractors were to be allowed 3 more weeks but earlier minutes had recorded that John Young and Benoni White who had been awarded the contract had to undertake that the work would be finished by 20 October or to forfeit £30 per week. The Minutes do not record whether or not this happened but the builders did have to wait for payment of the balance of the contract money until completion of the work. In November the Board was told that the new house would be ready by 21 December with the exception of the sick and lunatic wards.

Fires were to be kept in all parts of the building and hot water apparatus put in use when ready to perfect the drying out of the rooms. Mr Waylen and Mr Baker gave their opinion that a board floor should be substituted for brick in the sick wards. It was felt that the room designed for the chapel and the dining room required proper ventilation other than the windows, and the architect should also have thought of that, but this could easily be rectified. Recommendations were also made that a small hot water pipe should pass through the strong closet in the Clerks room and a small ventilating pipe carried through the ceiling to ensure books and papers were kept dry – again, fortunately, it was agreed by the contractors that this could be done at a trifling cost. It was also suggested that a tank be constructed in the men's yard to contain the large quantities of rain water from the roofs so it was not wasted and could also save soap in washing. Estimates were to be obtained for 'stoning' the yards so that water was carried to the gratings and thus prevent damp affecting the floors and foundations. It later transpired there were all sorts of problems for disposal of sewage. From this it would appear that the architect, Clerk of Works and Contractors had not anticipated many possible omissions and problems.

Although it is not recorded in the Minutes it looks as if there were some problem on the site with trespassers as the Committee had recommended that 'persons should immediately be employed to look after and protect the building from wilful damage'. David Lewis was employed to look after the house by day and night and to assist in moving the furniture with William Bennett as his assistant.

By the end of December a great many more defects were found in the building. Snow had come through the slates and ventilators and most of the windows. Fastenings of the windows were incomplete. There were no doors to the garden, without which the separated wall was useless. Almost all the locks, particularly the iron latches, were very weak and defective. The Board did not know whether the defects and omissions were to be attributed to the builders but if so they should be called upon to rectify them. If not their fault, it must be the architect's for imperfect specifications. A letter was sent to the architect about the defects and requiring his immediate personal attention.

THE MOVE
1836
On 20 December the furniture and 132 paupers had been removed to the new Workhouse.

1837
Colonel A'Court reported to the Poor Law Commissioners that the new Workhouse in the Devizes Union was in a fit state to receive the inmates. He was therefore recommending that the Commissioners should now order that all outdoor relief to the able bodied should be prohibited for all paupers in the Union, this to take effect from 1 May. An alarm bell was ordered to be purchased, the weight of which to be

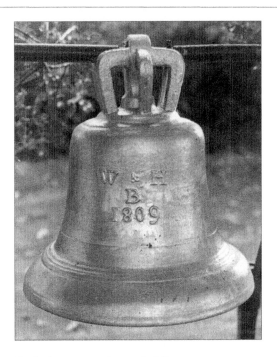

Bell which announced arrival of doctor, time to get up etc.

about 20lbs. John Slade was paid £14.1.6d. A photograph exists of a
bell which was hung at the front lawn of the building up to the 1960s
but as it has the date 1809 on it this cannot be the same bell purchased
in 1837 − it has not been possible to find where this 1809 bell went
when the hospital closed.

Several Guardians expressed their dissatisfaction with the new
House and again wanted the liability for this to be considered.

The architect had attended and agreed to instruct the
Contractors to sort out the many problems including the defective
state of the fastenings of the doors and windows. By 28 March the
Visiting Committee reported that the House was as clean as it could
be considering that workmen were still employed in it.

On 6 June it was resolved that two iron gates with stone pillars
were to be erected at the entrance. Joseph Holloway was awarded the
contract, his quote was £23.10.0. The base of these pillars is all that is
left of the front entrance to the site to-day.

IMPROVEMENTS AND CHANGES THROUGH THE YEARS

1839

October. A ward and sleeping room was to be provided for bad conduct inmates and women with bastard children.

A partition was to be erected in the boy's sleeping room with a close stool in it (a container at sitting height with an enclosed chamber pot) and a bell to be put on the stairs leading to the nurse's sleeping rooms. The door of the boys sleeping room were to be locked to prevent communication between these rooms.

1875

27 August. The Local Government Inspector called attention to the stony state of the yards. The Master was directed to remedy this.

1878

23 April. A letter was received from the Local Government Board directing that the Guardians should provide separate bathrooms for each sex and that a proper disinfecting apparatus was needed. The present usage was unsuitable unless extraordinary care was taken and was calculated to spread infection.

In July it was reported that work had been carried out for fire prevention and an annual payment of £1 was to be made for the flushing of pipes and hydrants. As a result the fire insurance was reduced by £1.0.3d. The extension of pipes and hydrants at a cost of £12.3.2d was also authorised.

1879

November – repairs to cow shed required. Tender of £3.15.0 accepted.

1882

16 May. Following the Government circular on fire precautions the House Committee considered the most effective way of guarding against fire in the Workhouse would be to extend the waterworks pipes into the Workhouse making them available for use in case of

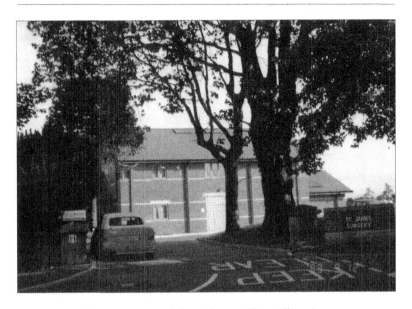

Entrance gates with base of stone pillars still in place.

fire. The Urban Sanitary Authority would charge only a nominal rent with a moderate fee in any case of the water being used to extinguish a fire. The cost was considered acceptable especially as the arrangements at that time were inadequate and urgent improvements were needed.

27 December. The walls between the young men's yards and women's were to be removed and the old and young men's wards were to be reversed. The old women's ward was to be made more comfortable with the partition removed – this would necessitate a new chimney at a cost of £5.10.0. The Board agreed to the expenditure as long as cost did not to exceed £35.

1905

27 December. Plans for a new male ward were to be submitted to the Authority by the Architect.

1908

14 August. A new floor in passage and cook house was needed. Mr Ash was employed to carry out the work for £8.8.10d. (All money

mentioned is in pre-decimalisation currency of pounds, shillings and pence, £.s.d)

27 October. The Master was to be empowered to provide material for a new fence at the bottom of the garden, the work to be carried out by labour in the house. It was also recommended that as considerable pilfering had taken place a notice be placed on the canal side of the garden warning trespassers.

21 November. Attention was called to the boiler in the tramp ward. It couldn't be repaired as it hadn't been fitted with manholes by which it might be got at and cleaned. It had become completely furred up, stopping all circulation. Tenders needed to be obtained as a matter of urgency. Mr Earle was chosen to supply and fix the new boiler for £15.18.10d.

1927

Gas costs were going up and members of the Committee thought electricity should be considered. The Board couldn't agree on this so a decision was deferred. A need was agreed later and tenders were sought. Information about cost from the West Wilts Electric Lighting and Power was considered and thought to be sound economically. This led to a decision to have electricity supplied to all the building except for the laundry.

1948

It had been suggested that the boot store could be used as a Physiotherapy Department after some repairs. However, the Master did not think the room was suitable because of difficulty of access for the patients. He suggested that the cook's bedroom might be an alternative. This was considered a good idea as it was close to the Infirmary and could easily be converted. Also the ground in front of the block occupied by 'mental defectives' could be made into an attractive place for open-air relaxation for the patients instead of a day-room or courtyard. Plans for structural alterations to the building with demolition of unnecessary walls and ramshackle out-buildings were discussed with the Master and approved in broad outline.

1949
New power points were fixed in day rooms for electric fires.

1952
Considerable rebuilding and decoration was going on in the wards leading to disordered quarters. New windows were being put in, ceilings redone, walls plastered and repainted.

1954
The new male wards were opened. The only criticism was that bed pans had to be carried past the duty room door. A few months later it was reported that the bathroom on the male side wards was too exposed. The yard door was at the end of the passage and there was a two foot gap above the bathroom walls allowing free access to wintery winds on aged, naked bodies. Recommended that the matter be treated as urgent.

1961
Recent alterations and decorations were continuing improvements made over the years. Major defects include a serious shortage of space for 'up'-patients in the female sick wards.

1972
Extensive repairs in progress. New flooring installed in wards 1 and 14.

THE END OF THE WORKHOUSE SYSTEM.

Old age pensions had started in 1908. The Guardians were reminded that they needed to agree and adopt a new name. Through the years this changed from Workhouse to Poor Law Institution, Public Assistance Institution, and finally to St James Hospital

By 1918 it had been decided that the system had outlived its usefulness but after that date unemployment soared, the war and its end having influenced the numbers using the Institutions. This might partly explain why it wasn't until the Local Government Act of 1929 that the real end of the Victorian Poor Law came about. On 25 March

1930 the Chairman referred to the fact that this was the last meeting of the Board whose functions would be transferred to the Wiltshire County Council under Part 1 of the Local Government Act 1929. Continuity would not be lost as the new Local Board would have four members from the existing Board. At the same time the name was changed again – it was to be referred to as 'Public Assistance' but the public were not convinced and still called it 'The Workhouse'. The National Assistance Act of 1948 can be said to be the true start of the Welfare State.

2
Children – Workhouse Inmates

To deal with possible privacy concerns, surnames for children both in the Workhouse and boarded-out have not been shown after 1908. The records at the Wiltshire & Swindon History Centre do show these names in full both in the Guardians Minute Books and the Boarding–Out Committee Minutes. The same applies to their foster-parents.

1837
The Medical Officer of the Workhouse was asked to visit the children of Mr Cook who was now in the Lunatic Asylum, and report on their state of mind and the expediency of removing them to the Workhouse.

1838
Workhouse children under the age of 12 were to be allowed to walk out in the country two or three times a week under proper care. The regulations stated that children could not leave the Workhouse unless an Officer was with them. Excursions outside did occur but only occasionally and in regimented groups.

The boy who attended the furnace needed a new wooden leg. The Master was instructed to procure a new leg for the boy.

1842
From this date boys aged 16 and girls aged 15 were to be moved to adult wards.

1873
9 December. The Board resolved to contribute £7 p.a. towards

maintenance in the Calne Orphanage of an orphan son of Charles Hutchins of the parish of St James. Two weeks later they also decided to contribute £5 towards the cost of apprenticing Robert Hutchins the second orphan son of Charles Hutchins.

1874

20 January. The clerk was directed to take proceedings under the Bastardy Act against fathers of bastards chargeable to the Union in all cases where necessary.

3 March. The Board agreed to take three of the children of Adelaide Pinchin, widow, now living as a servant to Mr Jones of Melksham, on her agreeing to pay towards their maintenance in the Workhouse.

5 May. The Board allowed William Long of Poulshot to take William Truman aged 11 years as a servant on approval.

1881

17 May. In the opinion of the Board it was most desirable that all fees for attending at schools, which the parents (not being paupers) are unable by reason of poverty to pay, should be met by a private subscription made in the parish for the purpose. Where this could not be effected the Board was willing to entertain the recommendation of any Parochial Committee on the subject, it being understood that any school fees paid by the Guardians would be a charge on the parish.

15 November. The Clerk was directed to inform the Local Government Board that they had taken into the Workhouse the two eldest children of John Webb (aged 35) who had a wife and seven children aged 11,10,9,5,4,2 and 6 months and was a labourer in receipt of only 9/- a week out of which he had to pay 1/8d a week rent. The taking of one or more child into the Workhouse was strongly frowned on by the Poor Law Commission and on 29 November a letter from the Local Government Board was received declining to assent to two of the children of John Webb being taken into the Workhouse on the grounds that it would be relief in aid of wages and would give an apparent claim for relief to every labourer with a large family.

The Secretary was instructed to see about placing Violet Smith in service. She was an inmate of the Union and helping with the children and had asked to be allowed to take up a situation.

1882
17 October. The Master was required to give the Relieving Officers notice whenever a child was sent from the Workhouse into service. The Relieving Officers were to visit such children at least once a quarter and to report to the Guardians in writing whether they thought there was any problem such as the children not being supplied with the necessary food or if they were subject to cruel or illegal treatment in any respect.

1903
There was a brief report stating that there were six children in the Workhouse and under the heading 'Infant Welfare' they were looking after Olive Margaret Brown aged 4, Robert Peter Crouch aged 2, Ralph Harding (who was to be returned to his mother at Marston) and Betty Pike aged 10 months fostered with Mrs Crawford, Woodbridge Cottage, West Lavington. The children had been visited and found to be well.

1904
If a child died in the Workhouse the death certificate would no longer state this as place of death but a nearby street name would be used. In Devizes this was 7, Commercial Road.

1908
On 13 October Mr Stephen Chapman of West Lavington had applied for permission to take Lily C into his service. Mr Chapman and his wife were elderly people and invalids. They had a son residing next door who had promised to look after the girl. He thought she would have a good home. The application was granted but the Minutes note 'On 10 November Lily, having been sent out to service at West Lavington where she was required to take charge of two old people, had returned to the House not being competent to look after them' (hardly surprising as Lily was only 14 years old).

1910

Having been deserted on 20 March Annie Elizabeth C was in the Workhouse. On 10 June her mother was reported as having returned to Bromham and it was resolved that she should maintain her own child. The child's mother, also Annie, was a singlewoman in service at The Firs, Netherstreet, Bromham. She appeared before the Board in August. After hearing her explanation why she had not applied to take the child from the House it was unanimously resolved that the child should be handed over to the mother and unless she took it away that day she must remain in the Workhouse with her.

1913

Discussions were again held about removal of children from the House following the Poor Law Institution Order.

1915

Five children from a Rowde family had been admitted after information had been received from an inspector of the NSPCC. The father appeared before the Board and asked to be allowed to remove his children. He had had his house cleaned and obtained a supply of bedding. After being severely admonished by the Chairman for allowing his house to get into such a dirty condition and his children neglected, on his promising that this would not happen again, he was allowed to take the children away. There is no mention of a wife – was he a widower or deserted father perhaps?

1929

Some of the children were sent far away from Wiltshire. It is noted that a young boy was to be sent to the Scilly Isles to learn gardening and he was to be allowed 1/- a week pocket money.

On 5 February a child was sent to a Home in Newport, Isle of Wight. Her father had written a letter asking permission to see her. The Guardian's reply was that he cannot be permitted to visit and the Home was advised that if the child was molested by him the police should be called.

Two gypsy boys named Mushie and William L alias C aged 6 and 3 were inmates in April and May whilst their parents were both in prison. When their father was released from prison the boys were given into his care.

Also in May the minutes record that George F had not taken his children from the Institution and the Master was unable to transfer the children to his custody as he had no fixed abode. It was decided to keep the children in the Workhouse for the time being unless the father should request that they should be handed over to him.

A letter dated 10 October from Beaking Sale Training Home regarding Ivy S child of Dora G, informed the Guardians that Ivy's grandfather had called at the Home and wanted Ivy and her sister Violet to live with him. There was obviously some alarm about this as the Home was told to refuse and not to give him the Worthing address to where it was proposed to send Ivy.

On 15 October the children of Richard & Dora G were in the Workhouse. Their parents had applied to have them back (the 2 youngest). This was refused by the Guardians but no explanation is given.

1938

The Pewsey lads were to be allowed a sports coat for when they went out, to wear instead of institutional clothing. These were supplied by local firm Giles and Gillett at a cost of 12/6d each.

1946

The Minutes record that the nursery children were out in the yard and seemed contented in a rather lifeless sort of way.

In her reminiscences of hospital life Nurse Peggy Dyke told that the nursery housed about 7 or 8 children. They might be there because their parents were ill but sometimes it was because of the loss of a parent or if they were illegitimate, had been neglected, together with other reasons. The little faces changed from night to night. It was the duty of the nurses to visit 4 hourly and to be sure that this was properly recorded in the report book otherwise they would get a telling off from the Matron, Mrs Balch-Ward.

EDUCATION

Early on there was a certain amount of opposition to the education of Workhouse children. Reading and writing, especially for female children, was considered to be of no use. The attitude was 'why would paupers be better educated than the independent poor'. Also the future work of girls was likely to be household tasks such as cleaning, needlework and in the kitchen. However from 1871 children from smaller Workhouses began to go to local schools and the numbers increased as the years went on. They also began to have access to books, the subjects of which were mainly religious and for moral improvement.

By 1877 opinion had changed slightly. In April of that year there was the first meeting of the School Attendance Board held at the Workhouse and by May a list of names was produced for the Guardians approval leading to the official appointment of officers. The Devizes Board considered that schooling would be of advantage to both parents and children if they were kept regularly at school from ages 5 to 10, the ages when they were unable to earn anything. Obviously the Guardians had their own ideas about what level of education was needed as in 1880 the Clerk sent a petition to Parliament on behalf of the Board against the intention to include additional subjects in secondary schools.

Teachers could provide a certificate reporting that the child would not benefit from full-time schooling. This report would allow them to attend school part-time and hold down a job for a few hours every week. The minutes show that some boarded-out children took advantage of this and gained certificates from schoolteachers.

When in 1873 The Agricultural Children's Act had come into operation it became unlawful to employ a child under 8 years of age in any kind of agricultural work but 8 to 10 year olds could be employed if there was proof of 250 school attendances during the previous 12 months. This was not enforced during the harvest season when many of the boys and girls helped on the farms and could earn a little money to help their parents.

1874

6 January. A circular was read from the Local Government Board about an Act of Parliament requiring Guardians, where out-relief was given to parents of any child between 5 and 13 years, to make it a provision of relief that education be provided.

Comments were made at the Devizes Quarter Sessions by the Chairman, H.A.Merewether, which caused some heated discussion in the town. Merewether had said 'that if a carter or ploughman could read the direction posts they were about qualified to make a good carter and a good ploughman but educating these people much beyond that was throwing pearls before swine'. His comments did not just involve paupers but all of the working classes.

1875

The previous schoolmaster had resigned on 18 December 1874 and on 5 January William Read was unanimously elected as schoolmaster but he resigned on 16 March. In early February the Local Government Board Inspector of Schools had visited. He found the children in the workhouse did not appear to be sufficiently provided with means of recreation. The Master's attention was called to the subject. On 16 February there were further details of the criticisms. The inspector had said 'I do not think the school is very well managed. There appears to be a want of discipline amongst the boys and the girls are not as clean and orderly as they should be. I found on enquiry that the children had not been taken out for a walk for several weeks'. The Board requested the Visiting Committee to enquire into the matter and, although not actually stated in the Minutes, the resignation of the schoolmaster was possibly caused by this adverse report.

In May the Schoolmistress, Miss Crabtree, had also resigned but it is not obvious from the Minutes why she did so.

1876

A new Education Act came into being in 1876.

27 March – recommended to parishes in the Devizes Union District that they should adopt the bye-laws for regulating attendance of children at school from ages 5-10 after which age some could go

to work provided they had a certificate from their school teacher indicating that full-time education was unlikely to be of benefit.

1877

In February the new Workhouse schoolmistress had resigned after just one month. It was decided to ask Mr Burges at the National School if he would accept children who were inmates of the Union and at what cost.

On 24 April it was agreed that the first meeting of the School Attendance Committee should be at the Workhouse at the beginning of May and that the appointment of Enquiry Officers would be brought before the Guardians prior to that meeting. Leaflets had been sent out to each parish in the Devizes Union saying

> I am instructed by the School Attendance Officer to direct your attention to the great importance of taking steps without delay for promoting the adoption of the bye-law under the provision of the Act. The Committee feel that unless this course is pursued the regular attendance of children at school cannot be enforced and the certain consequence will be that that instead of a child being released at 10 years of age from school attendance (which they probably will be if regularity of attendance is secured) they will be obliged to remain at school and precluded from employment until they are 12 and possibly up to 14 years of age, to the great injury of the parents on whom the cost of their maintenance will be thrown. The proposed bye-laws impose no restriction upon employment and the sole object is to enforce regularity of attendance at school from the age of 5 upwards until the children can obtain certificates enabling them to be employed. The Committee believe this course will be in every respect beneficial to the parents and children by freeing the latter from school and rendering them capable of employment at the earliest possible period.

1893

The school leaving age was 11 at this date and increased to 12 in 1899 and 14 in 1918.

1918

The Guardians' attention was drawn to the desirability of making full use of Certified Schools where they had separate children's accommodation and were registered under the Poor Law (Certified Schools) Act 1862. At that time there was no great margin of accommodation available but an attached list gave information about schools with an appreciable number of spare beds. This list of schools includes none in Wiltshire, the nearest ones were two in Southampton, two in Bath and one in Romsey.

BAPTISM OF CHILDREN IN THE WORKHOUSE

A detailed register of baptisms in the Workhouse is also held at the Wiltshire & Swindon History Centre. This starts in April 1871 and finishes in June 1932. The details include date of child's baptism, parent's name(s), abode, profession (many of the entries just say 'single woman' in this column unless the father's name is given when his work is listed) and by whom the ceremony was performed. Some of the early entries also include the child's date of birth. Although the bulk of the names have the 'single woman' entry against them there are also husbands' names on occasion – presumably the lady either needed medical attention or the family were on hard times, had perhaps separated or she may have died. The triplets born in 1909 are included in the register as well as the son of the Master and Matron (Hassall) in 1880.

3

Children – Boarded-Out
Boarding-out Minutes 1910–
1927

The following items are just a very small sample of the reports shown in the Minutes for the Devizes Union which give a detailed insight into the life of pauper children.

Marjorie B and Gladys B aged 13 and 10 to be fostered in Church Row, Devizes. In March 1910 payment for their keep was to rise from 3/- to 4/- per week. As Marjorie was nearly 14 and would be going into service once a situation had been found for her, the Board would provide her with an outfit.

In September 1911 Gladys was still at Church Row but by June 1912 the foster mother had moved from Devizes to Frome and had taken the child with her despite the Guardians' order that she should hand the child over to the Master of the Workhouse. She was requested to attend a meeting with the Guardians to explain her actions. On questioning she explained that she had a good home, better than when she was in Devizes, and wished to keep the child. The Committee resolved not to take any action and decided she could keep the child, but must send a half-yearly report.

Gladys C & Florence Lilian H. On 24 October 1913 the Guardians had parental control for Florence. A known foster mother would take her as she was losing another child who had been found a place at Stoke Park Colony. She understood there was some problem owing to a defect in the child but was told the trouble was over. In May 1914 Florence went to a new foster mother together with Gladys C who was aged 9. Each at 4/- per week.

In October 1916 Mrs Awdry (one of the lady visitors on the Boarding-out Committee) reported that the foster parents had informed her that recently the children had returned from school with bruises on them which she understood was the result of being punished by the school mistress of Worton. This was to be investigated. On 17 November the Rev. Campbell of Worton suggested the Committee go direct to the Head Mistress of Worton School. The Committee informed him that they could not do that and again requested he investigate the complaint of the child being bruised. In January 1917 the Rev. Campbell sent a long report made to him in writing by the teacher involved. It had been said that Florence had a bruise on her forehead. The foster parent stated that Gladys did not have a bruise which the child confirmed. The teacher reported she remembered the incident well. In August the upper class was in the yard to read in the open air, sitting at two desks and herself in a chair. The children read the same paragraph three times, each time making the same careless errors so she said 'Oh, Gladys, come and stand by me and I will go over the paragraphs with you. She did not come close enough for me to look over her book so I took hold of her arm, (rather impatiently she owned) and pulled her closer. No punishment was given or intended. The girl afterwards told her she had a bruise where she had 'grabbed' her so evidently the grip was stronger than she knew or intended'. The Committee accepted the report given.

In July 1918 Gladys was causing some trouble and anxiety by pilfering and untruthfulness with symptoms of moral weakness and she needed watching. Special training in a suitable home was suggested but it was felt better to leave for the present and await further reports. Satisfactory reports were later received by the Board stating that her educational progress created the opinion that her application and industry at her lessons entitled her to special consideration with a view to assisting her advancement. Enquiries were made about a free place at the Secondary School. By the end of May 1919 there were even more satisfactory reports saying that Gladys showed promise in conduct and ability. The Committee therefore were hoping to find her a suitable place in an office where she might find scope for advancement. This obviously did not work out as in July of the same year new efforts were made to get her an opening for learning dressmaking as she showed special aptitude for this. All attempts failed so it was recommended that she stayed with her foster parents until a place was found for her although in the words of the Minutes 'Gladys had proved to be one of the most satisfactory cases the Committee had under their supervision and they had confidence she would do well'.

Their optimism proved incorrect and Gladys, having failed to give satisfaction at Melksham where she had been found a situation, again went back to her foster mother. In October 1919 she was noted as having reached school leaving age and therefore should be found a suitable situation, preferably as a nurse-maid.

The Committee evidently tried to keep children of the same family together. On 26 March 1910 sisters **Caroline Louise C and Ethel Maud C** aged 11 and 6 who were under the Guardians' control were needing to be fostered-out. An Easterton lady had offered to take both girls. Mrs Awdry was requested to visit and inspect the home. If suitable then 4/- per week per child would be allowed with the foster-parent required to enter into the usual undertaking. Later she said she was unwilling to take the children at the above amount per week which included boots. As she was considered to be a very suitable foster parent payment was increased to 4/6d per week and this was accepted. The children went to their foster home in July and were still there in September 1911. In February 1913 Caroline went into service with Mrs Blackwell of Avington Rectory, Hungerford as a domestic servant (the Union provided her with an outfit which cost £3.8.5d) but she was sent back on 12 April to her foster parent who was asked to keep her until another situation was found. Reason for her return - she did not keep herself clean. By 18 July 1913 a new post had been found at Weston Super Mare but she was back in the Workhouse by November 1914. It was decided to send her to The Diocesan Refuge Home at Salisbury. However, by the end of January 1915 a pregnant Caroline was back in the Workhouse from the Salisbury Home and expecting to be confined in March or April. It was proposed she should be sent to a home where she would be taken with her child until she arrived at the age of 18 years when she would pass out of the Boards control. The Board voted on this and by ten votes to four decided she should be re-admitted to the Devizes Union Workhouse. In February 1915 it was recommended that Caroline go as soon as possible to Hope Lodge Rescue Home, Handsworth, Birmingham, to start her on a respectable course of life instead of being a permanent inmate and charge. She would be kept usefully employed in the Home and could eventually be placed in domestic service. This never happened as Caroline was examined by the Medical Officer and, although there were insufficient grounds to certify her as insane as some had suggested, the Committee evidently did not think she was suitable for this placement and they agreed not to send her although the vote was fairly close.

In January 1914 her sister, Ethel, was suffering from an inflammation of the eye and needed to be treated by the Medical Officer (Dr Lush) so he could decide if further treatment was required. In June a letter was read disclosing that Ethel had told the most extraordinary tales which were all untrue. Her foster mother was in bad health, could not leave the house and could no longer control her. Ethel had not been to school for three weeks due to some sores on her neck. It was decided by the Board that she should be brought back to the House and sent somewhere she could receive some appropriate training.

On 29 October 1915 Ethel had returned to the House. Arrangements were made for her admission to the St Monica's Home, Croydon.

Frederick C was aged 10 in June 1911 when the Guardians had parental control and recommended he be boarded-out but they were having difficulty in finding him a home.

One offer to take him could not be allowed as the lady already had two children in her house for reward.

In November 1911, as she was leaving Easterton for a larger house in Market Lavington, a known foster mother said that she would like another child in addition to the two children she already had. A third child was not allowed unless of the same family. Fred, aged 10, was available (he was at the time still in the Workhouse). After one month with his sisters (Caroline Louise and Ethel Maud) a request was made by the foster mother to keep him. This was granted for another four weeks when the Board would decide. Outcome – he was allowed to stay.

It was noted on 25 April 1913 that his eyes needed testing as he had a definite squint.

By November 1914, when he had reached the age of 13, Frederick had become too much for the foster mother - she could not control him and he had also started staying out late.

The Board decided to apply to the Church of England Home for Waifs and Strays.

January 1915 – places were available at Hedgerley Court Farm near Farnham Royal, Bucks. In early January Frederick was accepted on trial by the C of E Home for Waifs and Strays. The full rate of payment by the Board was required.

Alice May G was aged 10 in December 1911. In September 1912 She needed two teeth extracted and she had a goitre – treatment to be decided. In April 1913 Alice was being seen by Dr Lush who said she was better and was otherwise strong and healthy.

July 30 1915, when she was aged 14, the schoolmaster reported that Alice had sat an exam for a domestic scholarship at the Wells School of Cookery & Domestic Economy at Trowbridge. The scholarship was for one year. Her result was awaited and after discussion it was agreed that if she passed the Guardians would support her with pocket money of 3d per week (in April 1916 it was increased to 6d per week). At this time Alice was boarded-out at West Lavington. She won her scholarship and the Board recorded that they would be responsible for any medical fees.

During school holidays Alice would stay with her foster mother's sister at Trowbridge and the Board agreed to pay 5/- per week towards her keep but she did go back to West Lavington at Christmas.

Edith Minnie G was aged 8 in December 1911 (some entries give her name as Ethel Minnie). The Guardians had assumed Parental Control in October and had arranged for her to be boarded-out at West Lavington in March 1912. In September, having 'decayed teeth', she was seen by Dr Lush and had two teeth extracted. In July 1913 her foster mother complained of petty dishonesty both at home and at school. The girl did not seem to understand and was untruthful. She was feeble-minded although neat, affectionate and useful. It was suggested she was a case for a Home for Imbeciles. The Board agreed that admission to a home for the feeble minded would be appropriate. On 24 October 1913 a successful application had been made to Stoke Park Colony at Stapleton, Bristol at cost of 1/6d per day maintenance. Edith was to be taken there on Monday 3 November by her foster parent.

Lily Louisa G was aged 7 in January 1915 when the Guardians had assumed Parental Control. She was the illegitimate child of Louisa Ellen G an inmate. Looking for a suitable foster parent, one of Lower Street, Potterne was found.

In the same year it was recommended Lily should be sent to a home for the feeble minded. A report dated 30 July 1915 showed the child to be incapable of remembering anything she was told. She could write but could not read. In writing she could form the letters but could not put them together in words. However, she was quick at anything to do with manual work.

26 January 1916 the foster parent wished to give up the girl but was willing to keep her until the end of the month until another home was found. The reason was the child's bad habits. It was suggested that Lily would be suitable for a training school type home.

On 28 July 1916 she was aged 9 and noted as formerly at Potterne but since 13 March had been living at the Shelter, 20, Long Street, Devizes. The Board proposed to ask the County Education Committee to bear the cost of her maintenance at Hastings and St Leonards Special Resident School. However, they doubted that the Education Committee would help if the child was resident in a Workhouse or Institution when she had been boarded-out by Guardians. The Education Committee would pay if the Guardians got permission from the Local Government Board to send her to an Institution. Cost would be £40 p.a. The Guardians had to await a reply from the Local Government Board who replied that it appeared most undesirable to keep her any longer than necessary in the Workhouse. The Master reported that the girl was due to be returned to the Workhouse the next day as the house in Long Street would be closed for a while. It was noted later that Lily had been receiving personal instruction there.

On 17 November 1916 the House Committee were of the opinion she should not be sent to an Institute for Mental Defectives. The child and the nurse caring for her were sent for and the nurse reported that the child was bright, did what she was told but was backward. The report from Potterne School about the progress of Lily said it was very doubtful that a foster parent could be found who would be willing to take the child. The motion that the original decision be upheld was carried. The Clerk was instructed to get in touch with the Matron of the Elizabeth Barclay Home for Backward Girls at Bodmin to see if there was a vacancy.

James Lewis H was aged 10 in July 1914. The proposed home at Rowde was not considered suitable. The Master of the Workhouse thought that James would be better in an Institution. Letters were sent to Dr Barnardo's Homes and the Church of England Home for Waifs and Strays. Barnardo's reply was that they only accepted boys suitable for emigration, at least 12 years of age and of good health and character. However the Church of England was willing to take him and he was admitted to Soudy's Home, Sampford Peverell, Devon.

Elsie H (also known as Bessie) aged 6 was listed on 10 June 1910 as 'deserted'. She caused huge problems for the Fostering-out Committee as her health and behaviour made it difficult for a stable home to be found for her. Initially Elsie went to her new foster parent in Estcourt Street, Devizes, after the Medical Officer said she was suitable for boarding-out. On 27 September 1912 Elsie had a bad throat and the Foster parent was authorised to call in Dr Raby. Elsie was quite unwell in April 1913. Her symptoms were a bad throat and laboured breathing when asleep, which were quite distressing to hear. The foster mother wished another home be found for Elsie as the care of her was too much. Miss Walton Evans (one of the appointed Lady Visitors) reported that she had recently examined the child and recommended that she be taken to a medical man for a report on her throat, teeth and spine, as she was not at all satisfied with her health. Another foster parent was found in Bishops Cannings who said she would be pleased to take her. Miss Fox (another of the appointed Lady Visitors) was requested to report on the suitability of the home and if satisfactory to hand the child over. All was well and Elsie went there on 26 May. In a letter on 18 July 1913 it was said that the child was suffering from great pain through not having her teeth seen to. Elsie was to be examined by Dr Raby again and if he recommended it she should be taken to Mr Parker to have dental treatment. The Minutes later say that she was successfully treated.

24 October 1913. A new home was proposed for Elsie at number 7 Dunkirk when the Bishops Cannings fosterers gave her up. In July she attended before the Committee as unfortunately the new foster mother also wished to give up the child owing to the fits of screaming that Elsie frequently indulged in but said she would keep her until a new placement was found.

In April 1915 Elsie had gone to another home but this hadn't worked out either and the foster mother said she was also sorry to have to give her up. She said the child was untruthful and could not be cured despite being punished over and over again. Other than a note that the weekly payment to the foster parent had been increased to 5/- per week the next entry notes that the Committee had been informed that the foster mother with whom Elsie had first been boarded-out, wished to have her back again – the placement was agreed. Hopefully this was a happy outcome.

Edward James H was aged 10 in March 1918 and boarded-out at Hawkstreet, Bromham. The foster parent had removed the boy from the National School and also from the Church of England Sunday School and this caused the Board some concern. The home conditions were investigated and it was resolved that unless the two soldiers, who at that date were stated to be residing in the house temporarily for one month, were withdrawn from the house and the boy sent to the National School and the Sunday School as previously arranged, then Edward would be removed from the care of the foster parents. A later report from the schoolmaster confirmed that the conditions had been followed.

In November 1926 **Rose Maggie J and Audrey Phyllis B** both aged 3 had been boarded out by Bath Union in the Devizes Union Workhouse. The children had been visited and there were queries about their baptisms and vaccinations as this information was needed by the Boarding-out Committee. Questions were also asked about payment by the Bath Union and what arrangements were to be made regarding medical attendance.

Doris Kate M aged 7 was under the Guardians' control in June 1910. She was placed at a Devizes address after checking the suitability of the accommodation. The foster parents were willing to accept the child at five shillings per week. Doris moved from the Workhouse on 18 July. The full amount was allocated, after the Medical Officer approved, because of the child's delicate and rickety state.

In October 1910 it was reported that she was defective and needed medical assistance. Dr Raby was asked to attend after the foster mother, owing to the child's defects, said she could not keep Doris. In early October she was handed over to the Master.

The child's mother, who was living in Woking, had asked to have her back, this was agreed and on 5 October Doris was sent to her mother

26 March 1910 brother and sister, **Elizabeth Jane and Henry N**, aged 13 and 10, were sent to their new foster mother at Lower Street, Potterne. By June 1911 the girl had gone into a situation in Bath and her payment was stopped. Henry's allowance was increased from 2/6d to 4/-. He was still at Potterne in September 1911.

In April 1913 the Visiting Officer reported that there was still difficulty in seeing Henry but that a good account had been received for him. On 28 April 1913 Henry's report from the Schoolmaster on his appearance and conduct stated 'good and progress fair'.

By May 1914 Henry was working for J.J.Strong a baker, in the Brittox, Devizes, but would shortly be apprenticed by the Wiltshire Society to a Mr Burden, carpenter of Potterne, a five year apprenticeship. His foster parent reported that her income was nine shillings a week from a brother and three shillings from the boy who for his first year would receive three shillings a week rising yearly to eight shillings per week for the last year. She requested an increase from the one shilling per week she received to two shillings per week until he reached the age of 16. The increase was agreed plus she was to have ten shillings per quarter towards repair and renewal of his clothing.

Ellen Louisa and Kate Florence R. Towards the end of January 1911 the girls were under the Guardians' control. When they were aged 11 and 9 they were found a suitable foster mother but she brought them back to the Workhouse on 19 September after just one month as she was leaving the area. It was then decided to send them to West Lavington.

Kate's foster parent requested an increase to four and sixpence per week as she was growing very fast and had a large appetite. The increase was agreed plus ten shillings per quarter for repair and renewal of clothing.

24 June 1910. An All Cannings family had offered to take some children. The Rev. Crisall was requested to visit and report on their suitability. If agreed, the two sisters, then aged 12 and 11, were to go at 4/- each per week. However, it was found that two of the possible foster homes were not eligible to take two children. One because she had taken another child and the second because her husband was a servant in the employ of the Guardians, making it illegal to enter into a contract with them. The girls were finally boarded out in Easterton. By 16 October a place had been found for Ellen Louisa at a training institution at Bath under the supervision of The Ladies Association for the Care of Friendless Girls at 3, Spencers, Belle Vue, Bath. Maintenance cost was 5/- per week which the Board agreed to

pay. There is a note to say that the foster mother had wished to return her to the Workhouse but instead it had been decided that she go to a training home where she would be fitted out for going into domestic service.

However, in January 1916 both Kate and Ellen were at a Home of Industry in Salisbury and were each to receive 3d per week pocket money.

John R, aged 7, had been recommended for boarding-out in June 1911 but by September he was still in the House. Two months later a home was found in Stert with a lady whose husband was an attendant at the Asylum. The foster parent was to get four shillings per week plus ten shillings a quarter clothing allowance.

In March 1912 John had an eye problem, a complicated condition, and he needed to be sent to the Bath Eye Infirmary for examination. He had about one twelfth of normal vision, one quarter with glasses. The diagnosis was 'irregular astigmatism'.

In June 1912 he was seen at Bath and special spectacles recommended, cost 10/6d. They were found to be of considerable benefit. On 28 April 1913 he was reported to be a strong and healthy boy with a big appetite. His allowance was to be increased from 4/- to 4/6d per week.

On 20 April 1916 an application to take him from school by W.Hamblen of Marden Mill was refused.

November 1916 John was again sent to Bath Eye Infirmary for treatment and fresh glasses were prescribed.

In October when he was 14 years of age, he failed the exam for Dauntsey Agricultural School (arithmetic) but the Guardians, after hearing that one of the teachers had taken an interest in the boy, thought he should be given a chance and it was decided that they would pay his tuition costs of £7.10.0 for 1 year.

In October 1919 there had been difficulty in finding a suitable home for **Stanley George S**, so no special effort was made to board him out immediately and he was to remain under the care of the Master. Later in the year he was boarded-out at Worton. In 1924, aged 11 years, a report from the schoolmaster suggested that being a sharp boy he should be allowed to sit for the examination for a free place at Secondary School which he did and duly passed. Before the Board decided to allow him to accept a request was made for the Medical Officer asking him for a report on Stanley's physical condition. The Board were not sure about this as the boy had 'certain constitutional peculiarities' (not specified) and therefore did not recommend him going to Secondary School but that he should continue his lessons as at present until old enough to be apprenticed to learn a trade.

In November 1926 the foster family had moved to Potterne, the accommodation was a great improvement. A happy ending for the child – in January 1927 Stanley George was formally adopted.

William W, aged 13 in March 1910, was fostered-out at Potterne with his uncle. In June the relative had called to say the boy was now entitled to a half-time certificate and he wanted to know, if the lad availed himself of this and was employed by him on his farm, whether he would lose the allowance of 2/6d per week he was receiving as foster parent. The Clerk was directed to get a report from the schoolmaster as to the boy's capabilities and whether it was desirable, having regard to the future, if he should continue at school for another 12 months or attend school as a half-timer. On 22 July the schoolmaster at Potterne School said the lad had already been granted a half-time certificate and was availing himself of it. He was of moderate intelligence and if he attended school as a half-timer until he was 14 he would receive as much education as he was likely to benefit from. The 2/6d per week was allowed for the time being. William was still with his uncle in September 1911 but the allowance had been stopped in January of the same year.

On 21 June 1912 **Edith Emily W** had decayed teeth. Dr Raby examined her and said one extraction was needed and 2 or 3 others needed filling. The uncle of Edith was to be asked if he would bear the expense of the dentist and treatment. It is not noted in the Minutes but presumably she is the sister of the William previously mentioned as being fostered out to his uncle of Potterne.

28 March 1913, when Edith was aged 14, she was offered a position as an under-housemaid with Mrs Awdry. This was agreed to by the Board.

ADMINISTRATION

Members of the Boarding-out Committee were to be appointed annually by the Board of Guardians. The first Chairman was Mr. T. W. Ferris. The duties of the Committee were to include finding and superintending homes for pauper children. There were a lot of forms to be filled out and sent regularly to the Secretary of the Government Board in Whitehall together with yearly returns.

The first meeting was held on Saturday 26 March 1910 with five men and two lady 'co-operators'. The Committee described how Mrs Charles Awdry had been given the job of visiting the children and making the monthly reports to the Committee plus paying the weekly sums to the foster parents. Miss Edgell was to do similar work in respect of children with foster parents in Devizes.

In early June the Committee went into the question of what cases at that date there were in the Workhouse which came within the definition of the Poor Law Act of 1891.

The Master reported the following:-

Orphans – Nil
Deserted children – 3.
Children in respect of whom the Guardians had assumed parental control – 4.

The children named were Annie Elizabeth C aged 3, Elsie H aged 6, Doris Kate M aged 7, sisters Ellen and Kate R aged 12 and 11 respectively and Caroline Louise C aged 11 and her sister Ethel aged 6.

At this Committee meeting there was also a lot of time spent defining 'Orphan' and the Board's responsibility for children under the Poor Law Act of 1899.

It was resolved, with the exception of Ann C whose mother was reported to have returned to Bromham, and who it was thought should maintain her own child, that if suitable homes could be found the children should be boarded out accordingly.

1911

In December the new Boarding-out Order was distributed. This replaced the 1899 and 1905 Orders. The main wording was as follows. 'To the Guardians of the Poor of the several Poor Law Unions for the time being in England and Wales and all others whom it may concern. Whereas by the Boarding-out order 1905, we, the Local Government Board prescribed, in relation to each Poor Law Union, regulations with reference to the boarding-out of pauper children in homes beyond the limit of the Poor Law Union also within the Poor Law Union. Whereas it is expedient that the Order of 1905 and the Order of 1909 should be rescinded, the Guardians of the Poor Law Union may board-out pauper children chargeable to the Union either within or beyond the units of the Poor Law Union provided that a child shall not be boarded out in a home within or beyond the remit of the Poor Law Union unless he is an orphan, a deserted child, or a child over whom the Guardians have parental rights. No child to be boarded out in the administrative county of London. Every Boarding-out Committee should consist of not less than three members and one third at least shall be women. In the case of any woman having no calling or profession of her own the rank, the profession or calling of her husband or father shall be stated and noted as wife, widow or daughter'.

Rules were then given for appointments, meetings, keeping of accounts, payment to foster parents, finding and supervising homes together with medical inspections, schooling and special provisions for diseased and weakly children. A book was to be kept with a record of proceedings of meetings (which was to be open to inspection), details of children boarded-out and regular returns to be made to the Ministry of Health in London.

The Guardians could, when required, appoint a woman as a visitor to any child boarded-out within the Union.

Births were to be recorded as legitimate, illegitimate and if born in House this was also to be noted. If boarded-out a record must be kept to whom.

There were restrictions on the number of children who could be boarded-out to the same foster home, for example not more than two children were to be boarded-out in the same home at the same time unless they were all siblings. If other children arrived then the boarded-out child had to be removed. Persons in receipt of relief were not to be allowed to foster any child boarded-out by Guardians. Foster parents must be of the same creed as the child. Sanctions could be applied for but were unlikely to be granted unless the circumstances were exceptional. No boarded-out child was to go to foster parents with a history of being convicted of an offence which rendered them to be unfit to be a foster parent. Also no boarding-out was allowed to a house or premises licensed for sale of intoxicating liquors.

It was emphasised that a child should not be boarded-out without a certificate signed by one of the Medical Officers of the Poor Law Union to which the child was chargeable, stating the particulars of the child's health.

Foster parents had to sign a form which gave details of their responsibilities.

Payments to foster parents were inclusive of lodging but did not include repair and renewal of clothing

Visits were to be made not less than six-weekly by a female member of the Boarding-out Committee. By 1914 there were two ladies on the Boarding-out Committee as well as eight ladies on the Visiting Committee.

Foster parents were prohibited from taking out insurance against a child's illness or death, or they would face withdrawal of the child. The foster home had to be within two miles of a public elementary school. The schoolmaster was to be paid not more than 1d per week and to report to the Guardians at least once a quarter. No boarded-out child was allowed to be employed in street trading.

1912

15 March. Reports were received for boarded-out children from Devizes Town Schools, Southbroom, Potterne and Easterton. All were noted as satisfactory.

1913

Although regulations stated that children under the age of 3 were not to be kept in the Workhouse and foster homes were to be found, this had not been achieved by 1915 partly because of the war but by the 1920s the number had decreased. It was also generally accepted that children whose parents were in and out of the Workhouses regularly created a special problem.

In July a letter was received from Highworth and Swindon Union, telling of a problem with mothers removing children from 'Scattered Homes' when taking their discharge from the Workhouse, cases of sickness and infection having resulted. This was referred to the House Committee for consideration under the heading of 'Women of dissolute and immoral character in the Workhouse'. Although the Guardians acknowledged the problem they felt it was impractical to detain women for 'immorality'.

1920

During the war it was not always possible to provide separate accommodation and in early January 1919 there were 3,491 children still in institutions around the country which required explanation. On examination the stay of about 1,000 children was only temporary or special reasons were present, so no breach of regulations was found. By the start of January the next year the numbers had risen to 3,084. The reasons given were the war and the strictness of the regulations. The principal points included the rate of payment to foster parents (in April Devizes had requested an increase from 7/- per week to 10/- per week due to the high cost of living – it had not increased from June 1917) and the requirement that children only be placed with a foster parent whose creed agreed with the children's. This regulation made boarding-out difficult in many cases.

The conclusions reached in the circular agreed that it was no longer necessary that the rate of payment should continue to be fixed by the Central Authority. It was acknowledged that the religious requirements were difficult but that the Minister would, but only in very exceptional circumstances, sanction a departure from the regulations that a child should only be boarded-out to a family of the same religious denomination provided the child attend the church and Sunday school of his denomination. The Minister accepted that all Boards would make every effort to remove children from the Work House and had been instructed by the General Inspectors to give the Guardians who had difficulties in meeting the requirements, every assistance in their power.

Under the terms of the 1913 Poor Law Institution Order, except for medical reasons, a healthy child over the age of 3 should not remain for more than 6 weeks in a Poor Law Institution which was not solely a children's institution. There were several schools in the area to which pauper children could be sent. There were two in Bath - The Williamson Girls Home and Training School and the Voluntary Industrial & Preventative Home for Girls. Around the country various institutions catered for different religious denominations, Church of England, Roman Catholic, Jewish, Protestant, Calvinistic. Boys could be sent to a training ship whilst there were also provisions for blind and crippled children.

UNDERTAKING OF THE FOSTER PARENT

To bring up X as one of my own children and to provide him or her with proper food, lodging and washing and to endeavour to train the child in habits of truthfulness, obedience, personal cleanliness and industry. To take care that the child shall duly attend at Church (or Chapel) and school. That in consideration of my receiving the sum of-----per quarter I will provide the proper repair and renewal of the child's clothing and that in case of the child's illness I will forthwith report to the Boarding-out Committee and that I will at all times allow the child to be examined, and the home and the child's clothing to be inspected by any person authorised for that purpose by the Guardians or the Local Government Board. I also hereby engage, upon the demand of person duly authorised in writing by the Guardians, to give up possession of the child.

In case the child should die the Boarding-Out Committee would be responsible to see that the child was decently and properly buried. Foster parents in return could expect reimbursement, if the child was not more than 10 years of age, of not more than twenty five shillings or not more than forty shillings if the child was aged over 10, for burial purposes. The Guardians also agreed that if any child, after being placed with a foster parent, be found to be suffering from any incurable body disease or from lunacy or shall in the judgement of the Committee be incorrigible and of confirmed bad habits, in every such case, upon the same being duly notified, cause the same child to be removed from the foster home and duly conveyed at the Board's expense to a suitable institution.

1913

Dentistry for Boarded-Out children. The Committee recommended the Board to adopt a rule to apply to these children the same as that lately made for the treatment of inmates. That is to say that the elected Lady Visitors be empowered to arrange for simple extraction but more serious cases were to be referred to the Committee.

In August the question of teeth was raised again – Lady Visitors were to take any child requiring dental treatment to the District Medical Officer for examination and his report was to be laid before the Board for their decision.

A letter was later received from the Local Government Board expressing approval of the Guardians' decision to obtain advice from School Medical Officers in regard to the health of the children and they would be glad to be informed when the Guardians' had made arrangements with a dentist. Once arrangements had been made it was agreed that a sum be set aside yearly to cover the cost of dental treatment. The Minutes show the names of the children who received treatment.

1914

In March boots supplied to boarded-out children were required for Ernest and Arnold H and Stanley S. It was recommended that the applications were granted but that, in future, requests for grants would only be acceptedy at regular intervals in April and October.

1916

In April attention was drawn to the increased cost of provisions and clothing due to the war and in April 1917 the Guardians had further requests for increased allowances. Because the regulations did not allow more than 5/- a week, a letter to the Local Government Board was sent requesting permission to increase the payment to 7/- a week and the reply was that it was permitted to do so up to the end of September but any further applications after that date would have to be made in writing.

1921

In January special medical and surgical treatment for children under the Committee's care was discussed. It was resolved to ask the Board to make clear that the arrangements with the Cottage Hospital be made (if it does not do so already) to include boarded-out children.

1923

Two children from the Devizes Union were boarded-out in The Home of Industry in Salisbury. Violet S and Ivy G and were said to be well cared for and receiving suitable training. Other children had been sent to the Swindon Scattered Homes.

Some children had previously been boarded-out in what were described as 'barrack homes'. This was felt by some to be demoralising and it was recommended that efforts should be made to get children into foster homes or Scattered Homes. The 'Scattered Homes' were usually in a residential area with a head-quarters for receiving new arrivals. They were mainly considered to be for short-term inmates and those requiring special supervision. Some of these became Council Homes at a later date. The accommodation could be in ordinary houses with not more than 12 boys and girls and the regulations said that there should be a charwoman employed and the house should be in a residential area with the children using a local school. Boarding-out in these special homes was considered to be suitable for orphans and deserted children. Swindon seemed to be the main choice when needing to find a home for some of the Devizes Union children if a suitable foster-parent could not be found. By 1923 there were three homes in Swindon and they charged 14/- per week for each child. The Devizes House Committee had visited the homes to make sure they were suitable and recommended the facilities, despite the cost, which led to the Board's decision to send some of their children to these Scattered Homes.

1924
The Ministry of Health acknowledged that during the war it had not in all cases been possible for Guardians to take actions necessary to provide separate accommodation for children chargeable to them. In spite of a reduction in numbers there were still too many children in Workhouses. Recommendations included transfer of children to certified schools, a fuller use of spare accommodation in 'Cottage' and 'Scattered' homes belonging to other Boards

1925
The question was raised about visits to boarded-out children by interested parties and also writing letters to the children. Reading between the lines it would seem that there might have been some expressions of concern from foster parents.

It was discussed whether mothers who were now married should have boarded-out children returned to them. The Committee felt that each case should be dealt with according to its circumstances and merits.

1927
By May it was noted that there were no places in the Children's Home at Purton but Swindon & Highworth Union had places in their Scattered Homes – Devizes sent them 4 girls and 2 boys aged from 3-8 years.

SOME DEFINITIONS

Child
Under 16 years of age.

Orphan
When applied to a legitimate child the expression 'orphan' meant a

child both of whose parents were dead or one parent dead the other being in jail, suffering from mental disease, permanently bedridden or disabled, being an inmate of a workhouse or being out of England. The same terms applied for a deserted child.

When applied to an illegitimate child, orphan meant mother dead, and a deserted child meant deserted by mother for the same reasons as legitimate (in jail etc.).

Foster parent
Person or persons to whom a child is boarded-out under the provision of an Order.

Institutional Relief
Relief given in any Workhouse or any other Institution in which, for the time being, relief by Guardians could lawfully be given.

The Boarding-out Order 1911
This came into operation on the first day of January 1912.

State of Health
The Medical Officers had to certify the child as suitable for boarding-out and confirm no contagious or infectious disease and that both bodily health and mental condition were good.

Responsibilities
The Foster Parents had their responsibilities and entitlements set out in detail.

The Boarding-out Committee also had their share of forms and reports to complete, giving the child's name, age and who boarded-out with. These had to be signed by a Committee member or Appointed Visitor. In noting the child's condition, attention had to be given to questions affecting the health, feeding, clothing and cleanliness. Detailed information was be given to cleanliness, order and general surroundings and especially to the adequacy and decency of the accommodation, particularly in the sleeping rooms.

These regulations gave the Boarding-out Committee very

detailed instructions which they were to follow and any requests to bend the rules were strongly refused.

The Wiltshire Poor Law Union Boarding-out Minute Books, held at the Wiltshire & Swindon History Centre, Chippenham, also include the following Unions: Alderbury 1902-1930. Chippenham 1912-1934. Devizes 1910–1927. Malmesbury 1915-1930. Warminster 1910–1934. Pewsey have an account book of payments for boarded-out children from 1902–1913.

4

Guardians, Committees and Staff

The Guardians consisted of the local Management Committee elected at the beginning of April each year by the ratepayers, although after 1894 the period had been extended to every three years. They were responsible for the financial management of the Union as well as the general running of the Workhouse with the guidance of the Poor Law Commissioners. They had to prove they were eligible (by occupancy of property over a certain rateable value). This meant that women had never been barred and by 1900 there were nearly 1,000 women Guardians around the country, although looking at the records none are noted for Devizes.

The first Clerk, William Edmund Tugwell, was appointed at a salary of £80 p.a. He was a partner in the law firm Salmon, Tugwell and Meek of Devizes and the initial Guardians' meetings were to be held in their offices until the Workhouse building was ready. The responsibilities of the Clerk were quite onerous. He was to attend all meetings of the Guardians and fulfil any tasks requested by the Board, check and examine all accounts, keep the Minutes and file all letters, papers and Bonds of the officers. His salary rose year by year and by 1926 was £225. This was higher pay than any of the other Officers, including the Relieving Officers.

In 1843 Edwin Sloper was appointed and he is noted as 'formerly a solicitors clerk now innkeeper of Devizes Green'. Aged 32 he had a past history as a Relieving Officer for six years and for the same period of time had also been the accountant for the parish. Other duties included acting as the Registrar of births and deaths for four years in the Devizes Union.

The Relieving Officer's duties included investigating destitute appeals but they were not in any way responsible for those who died of starvation or weather as it was not the job of the Officer to seek out those in need of help. On application for help the enquiries he would have to make included state of health, ability to work and family responsibilities. The officers had to attend the Guardians' meetings to make reports on the visits they made to paupers actually receiving out-relief.

1877

On 27 March the Board was re-appointed. The Board granted to the Clerk an extra £10 –this was the usual amount allowed to him for conducting the election of Guardians. W.Meek was unanimously elected as Chairman with W.Stratton as Vice Chairman.

A list of Guardians in 1878-9 showed a total of 37 for the 28 parishes in the Devizes Union.

1878

F.M.Lush appointed as Clerk

1908

Committee members – Chairman D.H.Butler, Vice Chairman V.J.Berry.

1910

Chairman V.J.Berry, Vice Chairman , T.W.Ferris. There were 20 other Guardians. Adams, Biggs, Butler, Cox, Eaves, Flooks, Giddings, Giles, Rev. Hill, Maslen, Pottenger, Robbins, Sainsbury, Sargent, Slade, Smith, Snelgrove, Rev Travers, Young, and Hussey-Freke who was a J.P.

1916

The intended resignation of the Chairman, T.W.Fern, was regretted and he was pressured to carry on for another year. W.Young was requested to take the Chair pro tem. Fern was not persuaded.

1917

The new Chairman was Daniel William Butler and the Committees were Assessment, Finance, House or Visiting Committee, Ladies Visiting Committee, Boarding Out, Children in House and Special Committee.

Also included were representatives of Wiltshire County Vagrancy Committee, Wilts Poor Law Establishment Committee and a Selection Committee which only met when summoned.

1919

Another Committee was added to the list – The Motor Ambulance Committee but not shown as still in place in 1924.

1926

Committee members had proliferated.

Assessment	12 Men
Boarding-out	5 men and 4 women
Finance	14 men
House Committee	8 men
Visiting Committee	9 ladies
Selection Committee	9 men.

1929

Three members had failed to attend meetings for six consecutive months. They were written to and asked for an explanation. Two gave good reasons but Mr P.J. Watts did not reply so his seat was declared vacant.

1930

The Guardians would cease to hold office after 31 March. However the Wiltshire Education Committee requested the Boarding-out Committee to carry on until further notice

STAFF

There is a large amount of information about staff over the years. Details can be found in the Minute Books, the Staff Register of

Officers and Servants and also census returns. This has made it difficult to decide what to include in this chapter so it is important to point out that what follows is just a fraction of what information is available.

The staff had little freedom and couldn't leave the House without the Master's permission. Even the Master was expected to be available 24 hours a day 365 days a year if an emergency arose. The Master and Matron did not have to be a married couple but many Workhouse Boards preferred to employ a couple to fill these posts. If they had dependent children they could be kept in the House with the Board of Guardians approval but the parents would have to pay for their keep. There were concessions, in 1840 the Devizes Union Master had applied for leave to have his child aged 9 months to live in as allowed by law, without any payment, until the child was 12 months old.

On appointment all staff members, including the Master and Matron, were warned that improper conduct meant immediate dismissal and if they wished to leave that one month's notice was to be given or money would be deducted from their wages. When the Master and Matron were appointed they were required to give details of previous employments and to provide sureties by naming guarantors. Most early officers had no qualifications but by 1914 more professional people ran the House, especially medical and educational posts. The Masters were mostly untrained and had to learn as they went along about discipline etc. Their main aim was to deter any that were considered 'undeserving' although they would have to justify their actions to the Guardians. On the other side they were also required to report to the Poor Law Commissioners if there was any suspicion that the Guardians' actions were against the law.

Although unqualified the Master had a huge area of responsibility for records, staff and inmates, keeping of accounts and providing statistics. In some areas, if the Guardians preferred not to get involved when things seemed to be going alright this could mean that Masters and staff could get away with too severe discipline. Thankfully there do not seem to be any examples of this in Devizes Union − the Guardians were actively involved, although at the same time the press and public were not allowed to attend the Guardians' meetings. The Master actually had the power to refuse admission to unexpected visitors to the Workhouse, even if this was a Guardian, but in Devizes the Committee members were encouraged to make unannounced spot checks.

The Master, described by some as 'The God', dominated not only the inmates but also the staff who received low wages, few holidays and had to live in with no pension to look forward to when they retired. They were organised in a strict hierarchy, the Porter was the most humble up to the Chief Clerk who was the highest paid, as he had the best education and also legal training. Training for most Officers was never widely accepted under the early days of the Poor Law.

The Union and Parish Officers Almanac and Guide 1860 outlines in great detail the duties and responsibilities of officers and staff, what qualifications they should have, their rate of pay, regulations for removal of paupers and treatment of vagrants, amongst a host of other information and directions that staff were expected to follow at all times.

REGISTER OF OFFICERS AND SERVANTS 1849-1930

Offices held include:-

Clerk to Guardians, Medical Officer, Chaplain, Organist, Relieving officer for Vagrants, Infant Life Protection Officer, Relieving Officers for each district.

Master and Matron, Master's Clerk, Infirmary Wardsman, Labour Superintendent, Porter, various nursing posts such as Charge Nurse, Assistant Nurse, Night Attendant, Imbecile Attendant, Infants Attendant, Lunatic Attendant. Ancillary staff included a cook, handyman, laundress and storekeeper.

Against the named staff notes have been made giving the reason why they were no longer employed such as dismissed, resigned, died, promoted, ill-health.

MASTER AND MATRON APPOINTMENTS

COZENS/MASLEN

4 January 1836. W.Cozens and Mrs A.Cozens were directed to be in the temporary Workhouse by Monday and to have accommodation

ready for the reception of 50 paupers but by the 11 January no paupers had actually been admitted as there had been difficulty in providing provisions before tenders had been put out and accepted. 25 April 1837 Mr Cozens is noted in the Minutes as 'confined through illness'. On the 3 July 1838 his death was recorded and the Board questioned whether Mrs Cozens could continue as Matron with the present porter to be Master as he was felt to be competent. Consequently in 1838 A.Maslen was appointed as Master with Mrs Cozens as Matron.

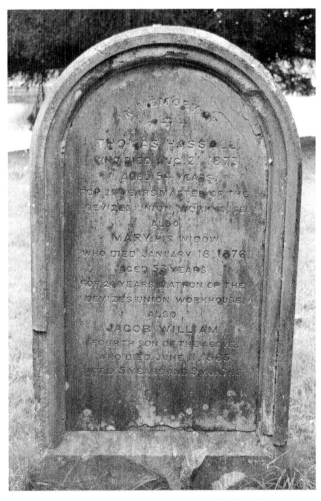

Hassall gravestone in St James Churchyard

SANDERS WILSON

Adverts were inserted in the local papers for a Master and Matron in April 1840. The advert excluded the usual wording of 'without family'. There were 13 applicants and the Wilsons were selected.

24 June 1840. Sanders Wilson appeared before the Board and stated that he, as the newly appointed Master, with his wife Martha, had taken possession of the House.

WILLIAM DAVIES

1851 – William H Davies and Mary Ann, his wife, appointed as Master and Matron.

THOMAS HASSALL

There is a gravestone in St James Churchyard. The inscription reads 'Thomas Hassall died August 2 1873 aged 54 years. For 22 years Master at the Devizes Union Workhouse. Also Mary his widow who died 18 January 1876 aged 53 years for 24 years matron of the Devizes Union Workhouse. Also Jacob William 4th son of the above died 11 June 1863 aged 5 years and 9 months.

HENRY JACKSON HASSALL

A son of the previous Master, Henry was originally employed as Assistant to Matron in January 1874 when his pay was £10 p.a. This was raised at the end of October to £45 but he was still noted as Assistant to Matron. At the same time the Matron's wages were to be raised to £55 provided the Local Government Board approved.

The Clerk recorded that Henry was 'confined by illness' and therefore reports in the Minutes were given by the Matron. The Clerk made numerous alterations in the Minutes crossing out 'Master' and 'his' and substituting 'Matron' and 'her'. This changed on the 16 February and the 'Master' took over. Henry was promoted to Master after his father died with his mother continuing as Matron.

In May 1880 the Hassalls had asked for an increase in wages – this was refused, the reasons given being the present state of depression of agriculture and high rates.

Henry resigned due to ill health causing permanent incapacity in September 1898. The records show he died in 1918.

MARY TIBBETTS HASSALL

Matron 1874 – 1898.

In the 1871 census Mary is listed as a schoolmistress.

January 1874. The Board approved William Jeans of Wilton and Thomas Mark Jeans of Salisbury, who were Workhouse Masters, to give sureties for Mrs Hassall's suitability as matron.

The Local Government Inspector had stated that it was illegal to allow the eldest son of Mrs Hassall to remain in the Workhouse. The Board arranged with her that her son should reside out of the House and that she should pay three shillings a week for her daughter who could stay in the Workhouse By August 1875 Mrs Hassall's daughter was assisting her without remuneration but three shillings per week was still being paid towards her board. The Guardian's resolved, in view of Mrs Hassall's long and invaluable service, that her salary be increased.

WILLIAM FEAR

The Minutes record that a vacancy occurred in September 1898 due to the resignation of Henry Jackson Hassall through illness. An application for the post was made by William Fear from Thakenham Union Workhouse, Sussex. He was aged 31, married with one child aged 7. It was proposed that the child be permitted to reside in the Workhouse.

Fear's previous employments were listed as:

Thakenham	Master from Sept 1897 to Sept 1898.
Camberwell	Porter Nov 1894 – Sept 1897
Greenwich	Porter April 1894 – Nov 1894
Reading	Labour Master Feb 1894 – April 1894
Reading	Porter July 1892 – Jan 1894

The Minutes state 'he has a competent knowledge of accounts, never been bankrupt, his whole time will be given up to the service of

the Union'. He had a security bond for £150 from the Poor Law &
Local Government Officers Mutual Guarantee Association.

His testimonials from Camberwell and Thakenham Union
confirmed that they were satisfied that he was competent. Fear was then
required to sign a letter confirming his bond and date of availability.

Similar evidence was required from Matilda Fear. She states she
was aged 32 and her testimonials from Thakenham & Camberwell
give details very similar to her spouse. The details of her previous
employment were:

Thakenham	Matron September 1897
Camberwell	Portress Nov 1894 to September 1897.
Greenwich	Portress December 1892 to January 1894.

The Minutes record that on commencing duty in 1898, they
were to reside in the Workhouse, his salary £85 p.a. plus board and
lodging and beer money. They were required to give one month's
notice of resignation or to forfeit one month's salary. Mrs Fear was to
get £40 p.a. and she also was allowed beer money.

William was Master from 1898 until 1930 with wife, Matilda,
as Matron. Work had apparently grown as Alice Long was employed in
1911 as Assistant Matron and William Trevor Fear as Assistant Master
from 1921-1930.

The Master was granted one month's leave of absence after a
recommendation from the Medial Officer that it was imperative that
he receive both change and a rest. It was agreed that he would receive
pay during that period of £7.10.0 plus his usual bonus

In August 1923 the Committee gave their congratulations
to the Master and Matron on their completion of 25 years in the
Board's service. The Master, in return, spoke gratefully of the cordial
relationships between the Board and himself during his long term of
office. William and Matilda retired the same year.

WILLIAM TREVOR FEAR

Known locally as Trevor, he was employed as Master's Clerk in 1921,
then Assistant Master in 1922 and also Storekeeper in 1923.

In June 1922 he had been given one month's notice so that new terms could be made on re-appointment. At same time the Master's Clerk, Infant Attendant and Cook had their employment terminated 'to bring these offices in line with other offices of the House'. They were to be re-appointed with the same salary they had previously received plus a bonus. William T Fear (Masters Clerk) and Winifred Henly (Infants Attendant) both accepted. The cook declined the new terms and left on 30 June

When his parents left in 1923 Trevor became Master with Winifred Henly employed as the Matron. She had previously worked as the Infant Attendant. Before he could take the post he had to provide a fidelity guarantee policy for £150.

MATRONS FROM 1935

Mrs Balsh Ward was employed as Matron from 1935 to 1946 followed by Mrs Nada Craig-Howell (with her husband Douglas as Secretary) in 1947. The Craig-Howells retired in 1974/5. Norah Marsh was assistant Matron at that time.

When Jean Yates, Matron of Devizes & District Hospital retired, Jan Sanderson took over as Matron, running both Devizes hospital and St James. When she left to become an Inspector of nursing homes the post then went to Daphne Lovell who unfortunately had the job of organising the closure of St James.

CENSUS RETURNS

These entries give an indication of the number of staff employed to look after the inmates although the paupers themselves would have carried out many of the 'menial' tasks.

1841 Staff   Sanders and Martha Wilson (Master and Matron), Samuel Stiles (Porter), Sarah Watts (Servant)
Inmates 149 (68 males and 81 females)

1851 Staff   Wm & Mary Davis (Master and Matron), George Cox (Porter), John Smith (Schoolmaster)
Inmates 214 (114 males, 100 females)

1861 Staff   Thomas and Mary Hassall (Master and Matron), Thomas Petras (Schoolmaster), Lucy Sainsbury (Teacher), Kennerick North (Porter), Mary Ann North (Nurse)
Inmates 149 (76 male and 73 females)

1871 Staff   Thomas and Mary Hassall (Master and Matron), Elam Jacob Pearce (Schoolmaster), Stephen Stevens (Porter), Mary Golledge Davis (Nurse),
Inmates 115 (61 males and 54 females)

1881 Staff   Henry Jackson and Mary Tibbetts Hassall (Master and Matron), John Giles (Porter), Elizabeth Underwood (Nurse), Emily Watts (Children's Attendant)
Inmates 162 (87 male, 75 female). This includes 3 blind, 15 idiot/lunatic/imbecile entries.

1891 Staff   Henry Jackson and Mary Tibbetts Hassall (Master and Matron), John Powney (Porter), Julia Ransom, Rachel Bond, Hannah Marshment, Edward Elliott (Nurses), Jane Slade (Assistant to Matron and Cook),
Mary Ann Burge (Schoolmistress).
Inmates 146 (80 male and 66 females)

1901 Staff   William and Matilda Fear (Master & Matron), Harriett Herring (Domestic Servant), Edward Elliott (Sick Nurse), Julia Ransome, Amelia Wells, Rachel Bond, Amy Pethridge, Rose Few, Henry Merritt, Charles Bowsher, Joseph Pocock, Arthur Giddings (Nurses), Clara   Martyn (Superintendent Nurse), Mary Parfitt (Needlewoman), Annie Few (Cook), Ernest Keene (Porter). Also the Fears' 10 year-old son James
Inmates 146 (81 male, 65 female). The numbers included 3 vagrants and 22 children.

1911 William and Matilda Fear (Master and Matron), James R.K.Fear (Master's Clerk), Sick nurses Julia E Smith, Nellie G Wheeler, Rose

Few, Mary Parfitt (cook), Heatherbell Smith (Imbecile Attendant), Alice M Long (Assistant Matron), Attendants – William Stour, John Clough, Alfred E Neate (Porter), Harriett Herring (Domestic Servant) Inmates 94, Patients 67 – Total 161 of which 11 were under 14.This number made up of 84 males and 77 females.

MASTER'S CLERK

1911 James Robert Kelway

1914 Henry Humphrey England.

1916 John Garrett,(pay 15/- per week).

1920 William George Quick (resigned 1921)

1930 Herbert G Looker (10/- per week + dinner each day)

PORTERS

1837 John Strong (died of Typhus fever late December 1837)

1838 William Masters, salary £18 per year with Board & Lodging

1838 Henry Hazell (died 1839)

1939 Samuel Stiles

1874 Stephen Stevens

1879 Benjamin Purnell (see chapter re 'Problems')

1882 John Durnford

1911 Alfred E Neate

1914 There was a vacancy for a porter but no applications had been received. A.E.Neate, who had left in 1913 for Canada and had returned, would do the job for a time and was therefore given a temporary appointment.

1916 William Stone. (Absent as he was a patient at the Bristol Royal Infirmary having had a serious operation. The Master was carrying out his duties for the time being).

SCHOOLMASTERS AND SCHOOLMISTRESSES

1836 Mrs Gray (another entry gives her name as Guy) pay 7/- per week

1874 A.G.Cape.

1874 Miss S.E.Crabtree

1875 William Read

1875 W.Browning

1875 Harriett Brain was the only applicant for the post but as she had not produced a testimonial Kingsclere Workhouse was contacted where she had previously been schoolmistress, to ask why she had left the Union. Reply was obviously satisfactory as she was appointed.

CHAPLAINS

1871 - 1874 H.Purnier

1892 F.E.Kyrme

1897 George Bird

1914 W.H.Weekes (died 14/1/28)

1928 H.A.James

DOMESTIC STAFF

1838 Martha Wiltshire (Servant)

1882 Charlotte Durnford (Cook)

1905 Clara Elliott (Laundress up to 1927)

1911 Mary Parfitt (Cook)

1911 Harriett Herring (Servant)

1920 Ethel Fox

MEDICAL OFFICERS

There were many Medical Officers appointed over the years not just for the Workhouse but also for each of the 5 districts. Just a few of the names are listed below.

Leonard Raby

George Waylen and later his son George Swithen Waylen

Frederick John de Coverly Neale

Charles S Rivington

Stephen Noel Varian

NURSING STAFF

1874 Mary Davis (Nurse)

1878 Ann Lucas (Night Attendant) resigned before qualifying period was reached.

1911 Julia E Smith (Sick nurse)

1911   Nellie G Wheeler (Sick nurse)

1911   Rose Few (Assistant Nurse) at £28 p.a. plus beer money of
6/6d per week. Promoted in 1914 to Sick Nurse.

1911   Heatherbell Smith (Imbecile Attendant)

1911   William Stour (Attendant)

1911   John Clough (Attendant)

1914   Emily Mayo (Assistant Nurse, promoted to Charge Nurse
1914, resigned Feb 1930).

1920 – 1930 Winifred Henly (Infants Attendant)

Nurses had to leave if they got married. They were expected
to cope with infectious diseases including venereal diseases as well
as looking after the dying. From 1897 the employment of pauper
nurses was forbidden although they could work under the supervision
of a trained nurse. The 1902 Midwives Act also affected Workhouse
confinements. These nurses often had to work more than 12 days with
just a half day off

OTHER STAFF

1874   Henry Kettley (Gardener)

1874   William Slade (shoemaker)

30 May 1882. William Slade had resigned as shoemaker, he being 81
and having worked for the Guardians for 31 years. Application was
made to the Local Government Board for a superannuation allowance
to be paid of 6/- per week. It was agreed this would be paid as long as
it was understood this was not a precedent.

1874   James Howell (Tailor)

1877   Emily Dyke (Girl's Superintendent).

18 December 1877 a letter was received from the Local Government
Board enquiring if any inconvenienced had been experienced owing
to physical infirmity but she was reported to have been in good health
since her appointment. Mrs Dyke had replaced the previous occupant
of the post who had resigned after she had been accused of misconduct.

1879 Emily   Hampton   (Children's   Superintendent).   Married
Benjamin Purnell (see 'Problems' chapter).

1882 Robert Howell (Shoemaker) employed at 2/- for every weekday he attended plus dinner.

1914 Alice Trumper (Organist). Left in July 1927.

In 1929 the Workhouses all over the country became known as Public Assistance Institutions with the Board of Guardians being abolished in 1930. In Devizes, in March of that year, the Committee was required to hold a joint meeting to consider the re-organisation of the staff at the Institution and they were empowered to act for the fixing of salaries and employing of staff.

Vacancies noted were Charge Nurse, Night Nurse, Assistant Matron, Cook, Laundress, Master's Clerk, Male Imbecile Attendant.

Mrs Henly was appointed Matron and on Dr Waylen's advice an advertisement was to go in the local paper for a trained Charge Nurse.

It was suggested that the post of Master's Clerk could be filled by a boy leaving school. He would be non-resident and earn 15/- per week but this was amended to 10/- a week plus dinner each day. A boy named H.C.Cleverley was thought to be suitable but one of the Committee proposed an amendment and a 15 year-old named H.G.Looker was appointed instead. An advertisement had gone in the papers for a Charge Nurse but no applications were received, however the Assistant Nurse post attracted 11 applicants one of whom was an inmate of the Poor Law Institution.

An article in *The British Journal of Nursing* in January 1914 gave details of the Poor Law Institutions (Nursing) Order 1913 which rescinded the 1897 Order. It was required that the Boards of Guardians should appoint fit persons to hold the office of Nurse, that a Superintendent Nurse should be appointed, and a Head Nurse if the number of beds for sick inmates numbered more than 100. The main proviso that affected Devizes Union was the regulation that no person should be appointed to the position of nurse unless he or she had had training to make them a fit person to hold such office. This didn't apply if an Assistant Nurse was under the supervision of a Head or Superintendent Nurse.

In 1949 the Medical Officer, Dr Varian, in his own words 'gave his heartfelt approval for the Master's request for additional fully trained nurses especially for night duty as there were more serious cases requiring skilled nursing'.

5

Physical and Mental Health, and Causes of Death both in the House and of those receiving Out-Relief

In 1836 the Guardians had enquired of the Poor Law Commissioners what should be done regarding medical relief after the formation of the Union, including whether the rate of pay for the Medical Officer should be for a fixed yearly rate or per head for a visit. Whilst a Medical Officer was appointed and required to visit the Workhouse regularly, initially the nursing care was largely carried out by inmates and it wasn't until 1897 that use of 'pauper' nurses was banned. The work was hard and involved long hours, often it could be 24 hours on call. As time went by regulations made it necessary for at least some trained nurses to be employed and the work done by Florence Nightingale in the late 1860s made it a more respectable profession and preferable to domestic duties. However, in April 1837 when the Master applied to the Board for a nurse to be appointed nothing was decided and at the next meeting in May the Minutes show that the appointment was to be suspended for 3 months. It is not stated why but at a guess the cost would have been a major consideration.

Medical Officers were appointed for each of the Union districts and also for the Workhouse itself. From letters to and from the Commissioners and Board of Guardians there appear to be lots of questions from medical men about payment for their work, both in vaccinations and maternity care, what their responsibilities were and which payments should be made by the Union and which by the individual parish. Although they were initially poorly paid, during the 19th century doctors gained in influence and were able, or tried anyway, to dictate what treatment inmates received. It wasn't until the 1840s that they were paid an extra fee for smallpox vaccinations, midwifery and some surgical procedures.

In October 1836 Dr Charles Hitchcock wrote to the Board and stated that he did not believe that his contract extended to all persons attacked by the present epidemic at Market Lavington unless they were paupers and whose wives or children were receiving relief, that is only those actually receiving parochial relief. The Board agreed to take into consideration at the end of the year the trouble and expense which he may have been put to by attending persons not within the terms of his contract.

Out-relief seemed to cause many problems. For example the Medical Officers for each district demanded details of payment and their responsibilities from the Guardians who in their turn asked the Poor Law Commissioners to give guidance on their powers to decide rates as well as who should be helped outside the Workhouse. It was explained that the duties meant that any person under their care had to be visited personally by the Medical Officer and that a named stand-in must be appointed to cover if the appointed M.O. could not attend. Also a report was to be supplied to the Board with details of any patient being treated including any seen in an emergency without an Order from the Relieving Officer. (The regulations said that the Relieving Officer had to provide an official 'Medical Order' for the District Medical Officer to visit therefore this provision was needed to allow for any emergency medical attention).

The duties inside the Workhouse were different. The Medical Officer was required to visit the House on a regular day and time as fixed by the Guardians. He would then see all who needed attention and give the appropriate medication. He also had to check each pauper on admission and classify if sick or of unsound mind. Of the latter inmates he also would have had to advise whether or not they would benefit from admission to a lunatic asylum. If a pregnant woman was to be punished the Medical Officer had to say if she would be able to withstand the allotted punishment. All children had to be examined and if sick advice given on their treatment with a suitable diet recommended. Duties also included reporting on any circumstances that might affect the health of paupers such as overcrowding and the state of the infirmary. The Medical Officer also had to set out the diet for sick paupers and report any deaths. In the Devizes Union a bell was rung each time the doctor visited to alert both the patients and the staff.

HEALTH AND CAUSES OF DEATH

Records in the Wiltshire and Swindon History Centre include lists of deaths in the Workhouse covering the period 1902-1939. This gives date of death, from which parish admitted, age, where buried, and if admitted as a vagrant this had to be noted. Also to be shown – whether the cost of burial was by parish or friends which would indicate who would be liable for the cost. There is also an Index of Deaths covering the period 1866 – 1902 compiled by David Kolle in 1993. The Register of Inmates from 1899 to 1932 can also provide death details.

There are some inmate deaths registered with an age of a few hours, together with infants and small children, but there are also a number of 90 year-olds. For example Elizabeth Bull of Rowde 95, Abraham Smart of Bromham 90, Mary Ann Baily of West Lavington 94 and Thomas Cooper of Market Lavington 90. In November 1888 it was recorded that Edward Hampton, an inmate of the Devizes Union House, died aged 101.

1837

In March there was an epidemic in one of the parishes of the Union. The Medical Officer was to receive an extra payment in order to deal with the increase in his work. The actual problem was not shown.
Some of the children in the Workhouse had 'the itch'. (This was probably scabies).

1838/9

In January the Medical Officer reported that there were several paupers in the house suffering from diarrhoea. He recommended that their diet be changed – rice pudding instead of suet pudding.

1889

An official table of deaths for the Workhouse during this year showed a total of twenty seven. Five were under the age of 5, six were aged 15 to 60 and the balance aged 60 and upwards. Four of the children died of measles. Other causes of death of the adults include pneumonia, phthisis (tuberculosis.), heart disease plus other unspecified causes. There is also one death caused by injury. This is approximately a quarter of the deaths for the same year in the Urban Sanitary District of Devizes which also included the Cottage and Fever Hospital and the prison.

1901

The Census gave medical details of inmates which included 4 with paralysis, 1 deaf and dumb, 2 epileptics, 1 blind and 18 imbeciles

1902-1914

In the last quarter of 1902 deaths in the Workhouse were 12. From 1903 to 1914 the yearly numbers varied from 16 to 34. In 1909 there is a sad entry of the death of triplets, just a few hours old, and buried in Devizes Cemetery by 'friends'.

1948

There was a suspected case of whooping cough in the nursery. The child was isolated at Chippenham but later returned to Devizes without having developed the disease.

1953

In January the mortality rate was high (as was usual at this time of year) with the Infirmary working to capacity.

1956

Four cases of gangrene. This was unusual. One died and the other 3 recovered following amputation.

1957

Protective inoculations against influenza were given. Although there was insufficient vaccine supplied owing to a national shortage the 'flu had spared patients and staff and they were not affected too heavily.

1959

The M.O. again reported an epidemic of influenza affecting staff and patients. Fortunately only one died.

1961

Influenza again – the epidemic spread through the whole hospital. Deaths were frequent, mainly due to secondary broncho-pneumonia and heart failure. Maybe this was why the M.O. needed a new table in the mortuary at this time (he reported that the present one was very old and difficult to keep clean). In 1949 he had explained that due to frequency of autopsies being carried out at St James Mortuary a complete new set of instruments was required. The Mortuary was also used for public and police cases.

1968

No epidemic illnesses in patients or staff. Inoculation against 'flu had been offered to nursing staff- nearly all accepted. No adverse reactions of any consequence noted.

1969

January to March had a very high death rate. There was no obvious epidemic but the majority died of a respiratory disease. A new disposable bed pan unit had been introduced which was meant to help with ward hygiene.

1970

The wards were always full and there was a very high death rate in January. For the January to March quarter there had been 44 admissions, 29 deaths and 12 discharges.

However by 31 December of this year, for the first time ever, there was no waiting list.

EXPENSIVE MEDICINES AND OTHER COSTS

1874

18 August. Because of increased costs the Medical Officers were to be contacted about the excessive amount of extras ordered by them for aged paupers.

1875

25 January. Mr Summer was in the Workhouse infirmary. The Board were of the opinion that he should not be supplied with extras unless he paid for them out of the balance of his pension which the Government declined to pay to the Union even though the amount received by the Guardians was insufficient to pay for extras.

12 October. The Finance Committee again called to the attention of the Board the large bills from Medical Officers for medicines. The Guardians decided that in the future the Medical Officers should give details of expensive medicines supplied, name of patient and cost in respect of each patient. The doctors replied that it was impracticable to give these particulars because of the time it would require. They suggested a compromise but this was not accepted by the Guardians and in November the Board specified that expensive medicines prescribed should be confined to Opium, Cod Liver Oil and Quinine. The Medical Officers were asked to agree. However they could not see their way to make any alterations in the existing methods of making out their bills for expensive medicines although another suggestion was made that arrangements might be based upon returns for the last 3 years according to the population numbers. W.Meek calculated that the amounts would vary from £1.10.0 to £30. It was then proposed and agreed that these sums be paid to the Medical Officers in addition to their salaries as compensation for expensive medicines supplied in lieu of accounts being delivered for these.

1908

10 November 1908. Expensive medicines £36.10.0, extra medical fees £21.11.6d

OUTBREAKS OF INFECTION IN THE WORKHOUSE

1837–1943

January1837. Influenza still prevalent.

December 1838. Diarrhoea. In May 1910 a Measles outbreak caused the Hospital to be opened at once for isolation and temporary help was obtained. January 1915. Influenza among staff. December 1918. More cases of influenza.

January 1919. Illness in the House, both staff and inmates but the actual illness was not specified. Possibly 'flu again. Reassurance was given that temporary assistance could be organised if necessary. In April there was an outbreak of scarlet fever. The patients (children) were removed to the Isolation Hospital.

From February 1922 up to February 1923 there were 35 deaths from influenza. In February 1923 there were 12 deaths, a particularly bad month for the 'flu. One death was 95 year old John Oatley from Rowde.

In April 1924 there was a confirmed case of Diphtheria in the Workhouse. The Medical Officer was requested to attend the next meeting of the Guardians to discuss this.

It is noted that in 1932 cases of influenza affected both inmates and staff whilst there was an outbreak of Chicken Pox in the children's wards. 1933, several cases of influenza in the Casual ward on the male side. In January 1934 six of the M.D. boys had ringworm, the number had gone up to eight by March 1943. There was a dysentery outbreak and Dr Waylen was investigating the cause.

1944/45

A Bromham woman and her 5 children were admitted on 24 October, the children were suffering from Diphtheric throats and they had been immediately isolated in the corrugated iron hospital.

The diphtheria cases were treated in the iron hospital because there was no room in the isolation hospital. The exact site of the hospital is unclear – in the 1886 Ordnance Survey map the fever hospital is clearly shown as opposite the path from Sedgefield Gardens to Victoria Road but on a later map the site is shown much further down Victoria Road (towards the London Road) making it look as if there were two hospitals in the area for a short time. This is possibly explained by an entry in the Minutes in February 1893 showing that the Guardians had decided to erect an iron hospital for small-pox cases at a cost of over £300.

In January there was a serious outbreak of Diphtheria amongst the Workhouse children. For this reason the iron hospital had been opened for the past 6 weeks for receiving cases. Because of the constant attention required during that period it was resolved that the nurse, Miss Rose Few, be granted leave of absence for 2 weeks and during that period her salary was to be increased by the sum of one guinea. On 9 February it was reported she was convalescent and had gone for a short holiday.

A letter had been received from the Local Government Board about the appointment of Rose Few at the end of previous year as assistant nurse, reminding the Board that they had not been informed what arrangements the Guardians proposed to make to meet the requirements which involved either supervision by a qualified nurse or special training.

The Board confirmed that an arrangement had been made with the Bristol Royal Infirmary to supply fully trained nurses in the case of emergency.

Mr Starkey called attention to the report by the Relieving Officer on Benjamin Davis of Bromham. James Taylor was directed never to suffer any patients to be unattended by the Medical Officer for more than three weeks, even in incurable cases.

1949
Outbreak of gastro-enteritis in the nursery. By 8 September this was at an end and all cases were convalescent.

1951
The review of the previous quarter was reported by the Medical Officer as 'the most difficult one for many years'. This was partly due to the

recent epidemic of an acute respiratory infection which spared neither patients nor nursing staff. Patient after patient had been infected, with broncho-pneumonia an almost invariable complication, and two patients had died.

FUNERAL COSTS

In July 1839 it was decided that the cost of funerals and coffins of paupers dying in the Workhouse should be made a parochial instead of an establishment charge, the parish to pay not the Union. However, looking at the death registers for the Workhouse this does not seem always to happen. If the next of kin were known they were to be informed and could arrange the funeral but often, because of the cost, it was left to the Union to arrange a pauper burial. This would be in an unmarked grave. The first entry of a pauper burial in Devizes Cemetery was for Edith Stonall aged 80, buried 16 October 1878. She does not appear in the inmate death index compiled by David Kolle so she may have been receiving out-relief. The Poor Law Commission's directions were that the funeral should be as cheap as possible, no bell to be rung and the service to be no worse than or better than the funeral of those of the lowest classes. Less eligibility even in death. The early Minute Books give cost of pauper funerals for adults with coffins at 8/- and grave 2/6d. A child burial gives same price for the grave but only 4/- for the coffin. In 1837 it had been ordered that funeral costs should not exceed 15/- unless the consent of the Board was obtained in advance. Also it was decided that handles were not to be provided on pauper's coffins. A one-horse hearse was to be provided for the use of the Union for interment of paupers dying in the House but only if one could be found at a small cost.

This desire to keep costs as low as possible meant that inferior coffins were purchased and in July 1850 it was reported that the coffin for Samuel Mead of Market Lavington was so poorly made it almost fell to pieces and had to be tied together. Funeral costs in early 1874 give details of arrangements for the funerals of Ernest Neate of St Marys Parish - coffin 3/6d, bearers and grave 3/6d. George Gray of Chittoe - coffin 7/-, Horse 7/-, bearers and grave 5/6d a grand total of 19/6d. Sarah Howell of St Johns - Coffin 7/-, bearers and grave 5/-. Freda Burton of Potterne - Coffin 7/-, horse 7/-. The grave for a still-born infant was just 1/-. Later notes specify that arrangements for deceased paupers should only involve the cheapest funerals with cheapest coffins although Bearers fees should be increased from 1/- to 1/6d. By 1877 the cost of coffins had risen to 20/- but in 1930 the cost had gone down again to 17/3d.

1927

A death in Devizes and District Hospital following an accident had led to the hospital having to cover the expenses and this had led to a request being made to the Relieving Officer for the District to undertake the burial of the body. He had refused. Although the hospital was legally liable the Guardians felt that the Relieving Officers needed to be given guidelines. It was thought that if the person had died at home the parish would have helped with funeral costs and therefore that discretion should be given for Relieving Officers to undertake burial of any person without means dying at the Devizes & District Hospital.

VACCINATION

1837

6 June. There were cases of Smallpox in one of the parishes of the Union. It was resolved that vaccination be adopted generally in the whole Union. The Medical Officers were directed to vaccinate the children of all paupers who applied for vaccination but not the children of those who were called 'second poor' (in other words those who were literally living on the bread line but receiving no parish relief or as mentioned in a Wiltshire Gazette report 'Working men just above poverty who are willing to dig and yet ashamed to beg'). An application was to be made to the Poor Law Commission for the Union to be allowed to vaccinate the 'second poor' children at the expense of their parish and not at the expense of the Union.

1881

13 December. At the next meeting of the Board consideration was to

be given to the appointment of Vaccination Officers.

1882

7 January. Fixed salaries could not be paid to the Vaccinating Officers. It was proposed that payment be increased per case from 9d to 1/-. The Local Government Board were to be asked if this was acceptable and with their agreement W.Glass and W.Douse were subsequently appointed as Vaccinating Officers.

MENTAL DEFICIENCY ACT 1913 AND BEFORE

The 1913 Act made provisions for the care and treatment of 'mental defectives' (persons deemed to be an idiot or imbecile often written in the Minutes as M.Ds) to be in newly established colonies and not in Poor Law Institutions and prisons. This caused a flurry of activity all over the country with Devizes being no exception. The new Act had repealed the 1886 Idiots Act. Its aims were for the care of mental defectives and making it the duty of Relieving Officers to supply information about the classes of people for whom they had responsibility to provide care. The Local Government Board approved of this and agreed that the Relieving Officers were to act as agents of the Committee under provisions of the Act.

Idiots were defined as those unable to guard themselves against physical danger, imbeciles as not capable of managing their own affairs or of being taught to do so, the feeble minded were categorised as those requiring care for their protection or the protection of others and, if children, were incapable of benefiting from schooling. There was also a fourth category of Moral Imbeciles – those showing mental weakness together with vicious or criminal tendencies where punishment would be no deterrent.

1843

In September the Board of Guardians received acknowledgement from the Local Government Board that they had received details of the number of lunatic inmates. This led to the query whether any of those on the list might be cured if sent to the Asylum. The reply from the Guardians in November was that the only persons included in the lunatic assessment, and not either in an asylum or licensed house, were idiots who it was considered would not benefit by being submitted to the treatment of an Asylum.

Classifications used included lunatics, imbeciles, idiots, feeble minded and insane, the main difference being that it might be possible to cure the lunatics and insane.

Roundway Asylum was opened in 1851 and before that date private institutions had to be used. This was not terribly popular with Guardians because they cost more than the workhouse, as indeed did Roundway (originally called The Wilts County Asylum for Pauper Lunatics). The Union was responsible for costs for any of their paupers who became inmates of a County Asylum

29 September. Entered in the 'Lunatics account' was the cost of removing Norah Hughes to the Asylum of 18/-. In December the cost for removing an unnamed patient to the Asylum had gone down to 16/-

1875

17 March the Collector was directed to obtain from the Oddfellows Society the pay due to George Smart of St James, a member of that Society who had been taken to the Wilts Lunatic Asylum.

1878

There was discussion about the best means of detaining imbeciles in the Workhouse without sending them to the Asylum. This was felt to be important because it cost less to keep them than to send them elsewhere.

1881

Isabella Masters, an inmate, found not to be insane so not to go to the Asylum. The Master was directed to treat her as refractory if she misbehaved.

1882

13 June. The Medical Officer reported that better provision for proper care of imbecile persons in the Workhouse was required. A committee was appointed to report to the Board and the next month Dr Waylen suggested arrangements for lunatic and imbecile patients. He considered that the number who required continuous watching was six females and two males, most of whom were in the infirmary. This number was not great and therefore insufficient to justify recommending that the tax payers of the Union should meet additional cost by the appointment of officers to attend to the lunatics and imbeciles. He also added 'In order to meet the difficulty arising from any exceptional or unusual pressure the Master should be authorised to call to his assistance the shoemaker whenever it might be necessary. If external aid was required the Master should be instructed, when it is feared that the strain upon him may continue for some time, to report the special circumstances to the Board to ask for some assistance during the probable continuance. If the Master had cause to employ external aid without the authority of the Board he should report this to them at the next meeting. Also that it was desirable that the Master, as far as possible and consistently but with discipline, allow the inmates who are fit for it, the opportunity of taking exercise in the Workhouse grounds at such time as he may deem expedient'.

1910

Names of staff in the register which is held at the Wiltshire & Swindon History Centre, who were employed from 1894-1930, include male and female Imbecile/lunatic attendants.

1913

On 30 January there were 24 'certified' inmates (9 males 15 females) with just 3 in the infirmary. The Committee was satisfied they were comfortable and well-cared for.

On 8 April the quarterly inspection of imbeciles had taken place. There were 4 in the infirmary but the others appeared in good bodily health and were well-cared for. Total was 9 males and 15 females. The Minutes also give the names of inmates thought to be suitable for transfer.

On 1 July there was a letter from the Asylum Visiting Committee recommending that the rate of maintenance be raised by 7d per week from 8/9d to 9/4d from 1 October.

It was emphasised that payments to cover maintenance were the responsibility of the inmate's parish of settlement whether they were in the Workhouse or a mental institution.

On 7 October there were 5 in the infirmary, the rest in good bodily health and well-cared for (the total of 23 was made up of 7 males and 16 females).

1914

In October the Guardians requested the Bristol Union to accept a 'lunatic pauper from the barracks'. It is not recorded whether he was a soldier or a civilian.

1915

12 January. The accounts showed the large amount of £490.8.11d having been paid to Wilts County Asylum

At the 12 January meeting there was a long discussion regarding the Mental Deficiency Act and attention was called to what was described as 'perhaps the most dangerous class of defectives'. The Committee should give immediate attention by, after enquiry, getting them certified as Mental Defectives under the Act so as to get control over them when necessity or urgency arose. Any such cases should be reported in full to the Local Government Board.

12 January there was surplus accommodation for 16 female imbeciles.

1916

Because Devizes Union Workhouse was accepted as a Certified Institution a payment of 10/- per inmate was allowed. Part of the House was certified as a home for the feeble minded and this is why the allowance could be claimed. It was stated that the Assistant Matron had the day charge of these patients and they were visited at night by a night nurse.

It was reported on 30 January that there were 24 certified inmates, 9 males and 15 females. As previously, the Committee was satisfied that they were comfortable and well-cared for. In the same year a report by Sir Frederick Needham reinforced this when he wrote – The quarters of imbeciles, 9 men and 14 women, are all suitable for their care. They were all neatly dressed and in good health. The imbeciles occupy the same rooms as the mental defectives and associate with them as far as can be seen without the least disadvantage to either class both of which are in very much the same mental condition. The rooms are very clean, bright and comfortable and the beds and bedding in good order. Weekly baths are given with fresh water for each person and occupation is found for them in the laundry and wards. There was just one criticism – there were no games or books.

In March it was suggested that the number of beds for female defectives be increased to 30. This was refused as the Inspector of the Local Government Board had recently visited and did not agree with the house reports that 14 women were defectives – he considered only 6 of them were.

A large number of people were housed in 'colonies', the nearest to Devizes was at Pewsey which by the 1930s had become the major Industrial Colony for Mental Defectives

July. The Minutes record 37 imbeciles in the Home, 9 males and 28 females as well as mental defectives.

1926

On the cook's day off the weak-minded made the meals (mental defectives were used as cheap labour similar to the way that paupers had been in the past).

1927

At the June inspection there were 32 certified patients (6 male, 26 female) chargeable to the Devizes Union. One or two were reported to be troublesome but most were amenable to discipline.

Frank G had been certified under the Lunacy Act but by September he had been discharged. It was queried whether or not efforts were being made to find a place for him in a home. In addition to being mentally deficient his ankles were so weak he almost had to walk on his ankle bones.

1947
The general heath of the M.D. group was satisfactory with the exception of one whose health, both mental and physical, was deteriorating.

1948
The Medical Officer of Health's report on 22 February listed 24 males and 15 females on licence from Pewsey Colony with 3 males and 2 females under the Lunacy Act.

The M.O. advised that more active exercise should be provided for the M.D patients but lack of space prohibited use of football or cricket.

1949
One M.D. developed a psychotic change. He believed he was changing sex and was demanding suitable apparel. The man was subsequently transferred to Roundway Hospital.

1950
On 23 November inmates included 2 women under the Lunacy Act, 24 men and 15 women under the Mental Deficiency Act and 1 woman detained as in a place of safety plus 3 men on licence from Pewsey Colony.

Conditions were considered unsatisfactory as there was little opportunity to segregate patients when they needed sick nursing.

1951
One M.D. patient gave trouble with rowdy and destructive behaviour and two gave trouble with sexual offences. They were transferred to different Institutions.

1952

In May the hospital was directed to receive certified mental defectives but the Committee considered the accommodation was no longer suitable. By 1956 only 12 mental defectives were resident. Dr Varian visited them daily and mentions them regularly in his reports to the Committee. For example in May he reported:

> All female certified patients have been removed and 7 males transferred elsewhere. There are just 16 certified males left, all over 16 years of age. The defectives now have to live upstairs in 3 wards with only 1 day room shared with other types of patients. The presence of defectives scattered around the building cannot be satisfactory. The chance of transferring them elsewhere should be looked into.

By August there were only 12 M.Ds and although the accommodation was still not satisfactory they were comfortable and enjoyed the amenities such as T.V., occasional coaching parties and escorted cinema visits. 3 were out at work and they contributed 12/- per week for their maintenance at the hospital. Work, apart from Occupational Therapy, was mainly in coal-portering and domestic work in the kitchen or wards – comment was made by the Board of Control Inspectors that they thought that the monetary rewards were rather small.

1954

All female M.D. patients had been transferred. The move for male M.Ds was in progress but not completed.

1957

The last 2 remaining M.Ds transferred. They were very upset as St James had been their home for many years.

1959

The Mental Deficiency Act was repealed and replaced by the Mental Health Act.

6
Settlements and Removals

Settlements and removals were nothing new. From Elizabethan times the parishes looked after their own and there were strict rules in place. Anyone in need who applied for relief had to prove their parish of settlement. Originally this had been place of birth but over the years, as people became more mobile, the regulations changed and became much more complicated. Women took their husband's settlement on marriage and children also took the father's settlement. Illegitimate children were regarded as having their mother's settlement but this might change - for example if they became an apprentice and length of employment in a particular parish was also relevant. Full details of the rules and regulations can be found in *The Handy Book of Parish Law*, published by Wiltshire Family History Society.

In the 1830s the new Act simplified the laws but by the middle of the 1840s new regulations were brought in which made proof of settlement more complicated. If an 'Order to remove' was needed then the details had to be set before two Justices of the Peace in the Petty Sessions.

Various reports have described the early Settlement and Removal Act as possibly the worst law ever passed by a British Parliament. There were punishments if someone removed under an Order returned within twelve months and again became chargeable. He or she could be deemed an idle and disorderly person within the meaning of the Vagrancy Act 1824, and could be imprisoned for up to one month or fined anything up to £5. The same punishment applied if a false statement was given.

The regulations specified that paupers in urgent need had to be helped before being removed to their parish of settlement. The cost could be claimed from the Union that accepted them and this is frequently mentioned in the Minute Books when a pauper is either being sent to Devizes or removed from Devizes.

In 1874 the Board received a letter from Lord Henniker about a Bill to be laid before Parliament to abolish the removal of paupers. The Board instructed the Clerk to reply that they were willing to co-operate. Although the Bill was passed, removals were still happening well into the twentieth century and statistics for 1907 show that 12,000 people had been removed that year. The principles of the Removal and Settlement Laws were still in force up to 1948.

1836

20 December. An Order of Removal was received for James Hale, his wife and 9 children from the parish of Bradford, Yorkshire. A report on 6 June 1837 stated that they had been sent from the parish of Urchfont several years ago to Yorkshire and they had appeared before the Board having been sent back. The family was discharged from the Workhouse, work having been offered to the father. There was also a letter complaining of Hale's behaviour whilst at Bradford but the details of his misdemeanours are not shown. The Devizes Board had admitted that his settlement was Urchfont and that they would refund any expenses. Consequently £5.8.6d was paid in March.

1837

30 May. Three paupers who were in Phillip's Lunatic Asylum were said to be chargeable to St Mary's parish but there was a query as to their parish of settlement. The matter was to be investigated and the paupers were to be removed or made chargeable to the parish to which they belonged.

1873

28 October. The cost of removing Ellen Gilbert to St Barts Hospital was £1.15.0

25 November. An Order was received for the removal of Sarah Weston from Plymouth Union on grounds that her husband, who had deserted her, was settled in the parish of Bromham. Order accepted.

1874

17 March. Jane Tanner, plus her 2 children, living in the parish of St Mary, was to be investigated and an Order for Removal to be made if the facts warranted.

14 April. An Order was produced for removal from the parish of St Mary Abbotts, Kensington to Devizes Union, of Henrietta Francis and her daughter. As it appeared the grounds of removal were incorrect the Clerk was directed to oppose the Order. This was later rescinded as it was decided she was entitled after the Clerk had reported in May that he had found her settlement was legally in Devizes and that the statement of grounds of removal should be amended and no appeal should be made against the Order.

April. A letter from the Calne Union asked the Board to accept Emily Jane Hobbs of Erlestoke without a Removal Order. This was agreed.

In May a cheque for £3.14.4d was sent to St Mary's, Islington, owed for Sarah Ashley and children under Order of Removal.

7 July. Settlement – Mary Jane Blagden alias Crossbridgeman, now in Hanwell Lunatic Asylum, was proved to be of the parish of West Lavington and therefore her settlement was accepted.

Clutton Union asked the Board to accept without an Order of Removal Elizabeth Hood and Fanny Cottle alias Flood. Later in the month the Clerk told how he had been in correspondence with the Clerk of the Clutton Union in the case of Elizabeth Hood and others. It appeared to be a very peculiar case (no details why) so he advised the Board not to accept the paupers without a legal Order.

7 September. An Order was produced for Mary Ann Giddings, chargeable to the parish of Lambeth, from the Surrey Lunatic Asylum to Devizes Union. It appeared she was settled in the parish of Great Cheverell. The Clerk was to make sure she had resided for one year without relief in the parish of Lambeth.

1875

7 December. An Order was produced for the removal of Ellen Jemima Dowse and her illegitimate child from the parish of Shoreditch to

Devizes Union on the grounds that she was settled in Devizes Union. As it appeared doubtful that her father, James Dowse, was not settled in Great Yarmouth the Clerk was directed to write to Yarmouth to make enquiries on the subject. The reason for this is not explained.

1878

Ebenezer Gauntlett's Order for removal to Devizes was queried. It had been proved that his settlement was not at Lavington as claimed. The Relieving Officer was asked to go to Southampton to make enquiries. He found that Gauntlett was definitely not settled in Devizes. Following this Southampton sent a withdrawal of the Order.

A few months later Southampton was again in touch asking about a settlement for a man named as Edward Wentworth. Would Devizes take him without an Order? This was agreed after it was proved he was from Devizes.

1905

A letter was received from Brentford Union about George Francis, aged 75, of All Cannings. In reply Devizes agreed to accept chargeability without an Order and would pay expenses of 3/- per week.

The Master reported that a man had been sent from the prison suffering from tuberculosis. He had been sentenced to 12 months for arson and was the second case now in the infirmary admitted from the prison. Enquiries were to be made to establish his place of settlement. A Bill was introduced by Parliament about the relief of persons released from prison. The Justices could make an order for the removal of a person and his reception in a Workhouse in the parish in which he had settlement. If this could not be ascertained then he could be sent to the Workhouse in the Union in which the offence was alleged to have taken place. If the Justices' opinion was that he was too ill to be removed to the Workhouse in his settlement area then expenses could be recovered. The Chairman, Mr Grant Meek, was not happy with the present situation where anyone discharged from Devizes Prison was sent to the Devizes Workhouse and the Union had to bear the expense, so he supported the Bill.

1908

13 October. A statement by the Relieving Officer reported that Edwin Arnold, described as a wandering lunatic, had been an inmate of the Three Counties Asylum at Arlesey, Bedfordshire, and was discharged on trial on 8 October. He had taken a train to Salisbury and from there had found his way to Devizes where, on the previous Friday, the police had got hold of him and brought him to the Workhouse. Several members of the Committee expressed surprise on the lunatic being discharged from the asylum and not handed over to the care of some friend as was usual in such cases. The Clerk was directed to write to the Medical Superintendent reporting the facts and requesting him to 'send for the lunatic forthwith'.

10 November. William Samuel Field aged 51, a pauper lunatic, was transferred from the prison to the Asylum. The Receiving Officer was enquiring about his settlement. The following details were found. The man was born 5 Oct 1857, Newcastle Street, Landport, Portsmouth where he lived continuously with his parents until 1878.

On 5 March 1871 he had been apprenticed as a boy into the coppersmith's shop at Portsmouth Dockyard. He was discharged at his own request on 16 April 1878 and since that date, although it was stated that he had served some years in the Westmorland Militia, he had not been in any place long enough to claim a settlement. The Portsmouth Board were asked to accept the case but they refused. The Devizes Board took the necessary steps to obtain an order of adjudication.

10 Nov. A man named Emerson and his wife who were on tramp had been received into the house, the man suffering from cancer. Their settlement was to be enquired into by the Relieving Officer.

1910

A woman named Pracey was brought into the House by the police and the Clerk was directed to enquire into her settlement.

In January St Albans Union were prepared to accept chargeability for William Hoy without an Order of Removal but suggested that it might be more appropriate that he be sent directly to a London Hospital. The Board agreed to this.

In early June an Order of Removal was received from the St.Marylebone Workhouse for a man named as Joseph Young. The Devizes Board decided to look for proof of the man's settlement and obtained a very full description of his life over the years from his sister Mrs Charlotte Bull. She stated that he was born on 24 February 1884 at Battersea, went with is parents to Northfleet then in 1885 to Devizes where his father, William Young, took over the post of canteen steward and where his mother died on 26 November 1885. He stayed there until April 1891 when the family went to Dublin where his father died on 7 April 1895. The pauper, with his sister, then returned to England (Melksham) he being sent to a boarding school in Walcot, Bath, then to Mrs Gabriel's boarding School at Calne where he remained for around one year. He then went to Mrs Pitman's at Coate, attending the Green school in Devizes for about 18 months till he was 14. He then went to his sister at Lowbourne, Melksham about February 1898 and remained there, except for two periods of about a month each, until June 1903 when he was at Mrs Lewsingtons, Bank Street, Melksham. Whilst at Melksham he was at Lowbourne School and then employed by a Mr Waight. He was also employed with his sister's husband at Mr Huttons and afterwards by Mr Colbourne. He left Melksham in 1903 and since then he had been at Belfast, Yeovil, Devizes, Yeovil, Weymouth, Yeovil, London Church Army Home and elsewhere. Relieving Officer Mitchell was sent to London to interview Young and ascertain if he was able to prove residency for 3 years at Melksham - if so a notice of appeal against the Order could be given. The case came up again at the 21 June meeting and the Clerk reported that the Relieving Officer had interviewed Young and had been able to verify the fact that he had obtained settlement at Melksham. With these facts before them a formal Notice of Abandonment of the Order had been received from the Clerk of the Marylebone Workhouse.

1913

On 15 July William Dowse, who had 4 children in the Workhouse, appeared before the Board and stated that he was unable to comply with the Board's order to contribute 10/- per week towards the maintenance of his children. He admitted that he was employed at the GWR Works at Swindon and was in receipt of £1 per week less insurance. The Board resolved to adhere to their decision of 1 July requiring Dowse to remove his children from the House and failing his doing that he be ordered to pay 10/- per week. Unless he complied proceedings would be taken. Early in November Dowse had sent a letter requesting that the arrears might be allowed to stand over until he got a home together. Because he had paid 6/- a week it was resolved to allow the matter to stand and be recovered when he had a home. The children had been admitted to the House under an Order of Removal from the Cricklade and Wootton Bassett Union but the relief was contrary to the orders of the Local Government Board and the Clerk was directed to write to them requiring permission for the children to remain in the House until the wife of Dowse was released from prison and a home had been provided to which the children could be sent. On 24 February the Relieving officer had visited Swindon and interviewed Dowse who had promised, in writing, that he would fetch the children from the Workhouse on 23 February but he had not come to collect them. The Relieving Officer was directed to take the children and deliver them to Dowse at his residence in Swindon. He did this on 25 February and handed them over. A letter from the Cricklade and Wootton Bassett Union was received saying that 3 of the children had been taken to the Workhouse on 25 February (the same day that they had been taken to their father) and as their settlement was Devizes for them to be removed as soon as possible. The Board were unanimous that the children should not be in the Workhouse and should either be delivered into the father's custody or that he should be immediately called upon to remove them and be prosecuted if he failed to do so, pointing out the background and that there was no destitution in this case as Dowse was working full-time. A reply stated that the children had been removed from Purton Workhouse and that the Devizes Board need not trouble themselves further.

In September of this year irregularities were reported concerning the admission of a woman to the House named as Mrs Hughes, and the following resolution was passed. 'Having before them the letter of 14 July from the Board of Control and the fact that Dr Rayment was unable to state some fact indicating Mental Deficiency as required in that letter, the Committee are of the opinion that the woman should be discharged from the House and moved to Pewsey Union as soon as possible'. They would also communicate with the Pewsey Board with a view to a boy's removal from the Devizes Workhouse to Pewsey.

1915

12 January. Some children had been admitted to the Home but as their parents had settlement in Reading that Union was asked if they would accept chargeability. Reading declined and therefore the children were to be handed on to their parents.

1919

In October the Board received a formal Order of Removal from Wandsworth Union for Mary Jenkins. She was chargeable to Devizes Union as she had lived for more than 10 years up to 1919 at 4 Avon Road, Devizes. It was agreed not to contest.

A boy, boarded-out at Potterne, was removed to South Stoneham Union.

1924

Devizes received these details from Cardiff Union requesting that they accept their request for chargeability without a formal order.

John Walker, properly William John Bundy, was born in Littleton on 31 March 1855 and lived with his parents. Once married he lived next door to his father at West Lavington until 1892. Since that date he had led an unsettled life, never having remained in any one parish for a period of 12 months. The Devizes Union relieving Officer gave slightly different information recording his date of birth as 30 March 1855 at Littleton Panell where he lived from birth until 1899 when he went to Wales and since then his wife and relatives knew nothing of his whereabouts. The Guardians decided not to accept chargeability without a formal Order of Adjudication.

1926

1 June. The Board discussed a non-settled case. The woman had been persuaded to remain at her home in Cardiff but had arrived in Devizes

with her four children and was living with her brother at Great Porch, Monday Market Street, Devizes. She had approached the Relieving Officer with regard to payment of non-settled relief. On inspection the accommodation was quite insufficient for the numbers. Temporary relief was agreed pending more suitable accommodation being found but failing this Cardiff authorised her admission to the Institution from whence she would be transferred to Cardiff. She was allowed 4 weeks to find suitable accommodation. By 29 June there was no improvement and no accommodation had been found. An Order for admission was issued and Cardiff was informed.

29 June. Alfred Maude aged 53. An Order of Removal for this inmate of Cardiff Poor Law Institution was discussed at the Board meeting. His settlement in Urchfont was confirmed but he had actually already returned to Urchfont and was living in his home and therefore was no longer chargeable.

William Fisher aged 40 and wife Edna aged 37. An Order of Removal from Lambeth, London, was received. He had settlement by residence in the parish of Rowde Within and also by parentage. The Fishers were receiving outdoor relief at Lambeth. Devizes Union Guardians were asked if they were willing to keep paying but the reply was that relief had already ceased. An amount of £3.4.7d was sent to Lambeth to cover what had already been advanced.

However by November William Fisher and his wife Edna were in Southwark Union. It was again agreed that he had settlement in Rowde Within. Maintenance costs were to be refunded and he was to be transferred to Wilts County Mental Asylum and his wife to Devizes Poor Law Institution.

1927

8 February. An Order of Removal was received from Merthyr Tydfil Union for a 50 year old man from Potterne (where he had lived from 1889-1896) with 5 children aged 13,12,7,5 and 4. He was admitted on 10 March. No wife is listed. There was mention of the possibility of Barnardos for the children. Devizes agreed to accept the family.

Jane Ackland aged 74 was an inmate of Willesden Union Infirmary. Her Order of Removal was suspended as she was bedridden, suffering from rheumatoid arthritis and too weak to stand the journey to Devizes.

1928

In April a Removal Order was received from Lewisham Union for a William Simmons aged 40, last legal settlement being St John, Devizes. The Relieving Officer was sent to London to investigate. It appeared that Simmons had not lived long enough to gain status of irremovability and it was confirmed that he was from Devizes. Therefore the Order was accepted.

There was an added note to this. The Clerk stated that upon receiving an Order of Removal it was frequently necessary for the Relieving Officer to make a journey and incur expenses whilst making investigation. From this comment it would appear that the Relieving Officers' did not get any refund of expenses.

1929

15 October. Alfred Fisher had been admitted from the Casual Ward to the infirmary on 18 August, There was an enquiry as to his settlement and it appeared he had last acquired a settlement in the parish of Battersea in Wandsworth Union and that since acquiring that in about 1892 he never had a permanent residence whereby another settlement could be established. On writing to the Wandsworth Union requesting they accept some chargeability without formal Order of Removal the reply was that a formal Order was required. This was applied for but Fisher died on the 29 October before it was issued but Devizes still wanted some re-re-inbursement for his care and decided Wandsworth Union should pay £1.1.0 for each week he was in Devizes.

Out door relief poster

7
Out-Relief

Before 1837 a tenth of the population were receiving Relief, this included the old, infirm and lunatics. The aim of the 1834 Act was to cut down the relief, both money or in kind, to people considered to be able-bodied. They were to be offered admission to the Workhouse or nothing. The choice was to go in to the Workhouse or to starve. Out-relief did still continue for some time but the 1844 Outdoor Relief Prohibition Act only allowed help outside the Workhouse in special circumstances. The result of this was that Guardians were still able to circumvent the Act if they wished and this meant that costs continued to rise. It wasn't until further legislation was brought in that payments gradually dropped. How this worked in the Devizes Union is well-illustrated in the Minute books.

1836

11 January. It was resolved that no relief would be given to any poor person having a cottage or other property except by way of loan and then only in case of emergency. No person occupying more than a quarter of an acre of land was to receive any relief except in case of emergency. This resolution was not to be put into effect until relief was stopped to able-bodied paupers having families.

At the end of February Relieving Officers were directed to 'use their best endeavours to visit the poor in their own houses in order to ascertain their state'.

At the next meeting relief of pensioners was discussed. It was decided that one third of any pension was to be regarded as a bonus or reward for service and this would not be taken into account when considering the amount of relief to be allowed.

On 20 July the Guardians received a letter from the Commissioners authorising monetary relief to out-door paupers as long as the Board of Guardians approved.

On 4 October the Urchfont Overseer attended the Board meeting and reported that nine paupers to whom loans had been made were to appear before the Magistrate as they had not repaid the money.

In November the cost for the 136 paupers resident in the House was £239.10.7d. The cost for the 1146 paupers receiving Out-Relief for the same period was £1,623.10.5d

1837

28 March. A report on a family named Cook was read. 3/- a week was to be allowed as outdoor relief, their friends having undertaken to look after them.

In the same month time was spent considering whether medical relief should not be an establishment charge but a parochial one, the same as out -relief. The Guardians sent a letter to the Commissioners asking for their sanction to make it so. Their reply was that the parish should bear the cost.

There were also questions about vaccinations of children of families receiving out-relief. A letter to the Poor Law Commissioners in June stated 'The smallpox having been prevalent in some of the parishes in this Union the Guardians directed the Medical Officers to vaccinate the children of every pauper now receiving relief. The Guardians believe that vaccination should become general and request authority to its being at the expense of the parish. The advice from London was that this should be decided after receiving medical advice. The Guardians were to take due care that the parties to be vaccinated were proper objects of relief and that the terms upon which the operation was to be paid for were not extravagant. However, because vaccinations were now generally included in the Medical Officer's contract this would make any extra payment for the performance of that part of their duty unnecessary. The Commissioners further stated that if the order of payment be by case then the expenses for these should be charged to the parish in which it occurred.

20 March. The Poor Law Commission confirmed their approval

forbidding out-relief to the able-bodied male pauper except in the Workhouse. The following month it was noted that there was violent opposition about the changes from the old system. There had been a request for help from a man of good character who was able-bodied and in receipt of wages equivalent to his labour but unable, by his earnings, to support himself and family. Some of the Guardians contended that the whole family ought to be ordered into the House. Others were of a different opinion and thought that one of the children should be taken into the Workhouse and the father permitted to continue to labour to keep himself and the rest of the family. The Board decided that one of the children could be placed in the House to help the father and sought the opinion of the Commission about this as so many similar applications were being made. The reply was 'Without wishing to interfere with any decision already made, the Commission urge the importance of adhering closely to the Order prohibiting out-door relief to able-bodied male paupers or in other words prohibiting relief in aid of wages. The Guardians' duty is not to sanction any departures from the rule unless under circumstances of the most peculiar nature'.

July. A letter from the Guardians to the Poor Law Commissioners asked about two men being tried for murder at Stert and three men for a rape at Etchilhampton. Could expenses be defrayed from taking up prosecution, the parties being too poor to engage professional assistance? The reply from London on the very next day said that expenses could not be defrayed from the Poor Rates.

1838

It was resolved by the Guardians that in all cases of non-residential relief the Relieving Officers be requested to bring all such cases before them each quarter.

1874

12 May. George Bullock of St James parish was allowed by way of loan the cost of a truss for his wife and the collector was required to obtain repayment by reasonable instalments.

The bills for bread for May show there was a misuse of bread tickets (which had been issued as part of out-relief). They should only be used once and the Relieving Officers were accused of not keeping a proper check on this. The Committee emphasised that accurate records must be kept to avoid possible mistakes in future bread accounts. The Relieving Officer responsible was warned that if his books were not kept in a proper state he would be called upon to resign or an application for his removal from the post would be made.

The quarterly accounts record that the cost of bread supplied to tramps was 2/6d. The total out-relief for January, February and March was £1,597.9.5d

On 18 August the Auditor pointed out that out-relief had decreased in other Unions but had increased in Devizes by £133.3.3d. The Medical Officers were to be informed about the excessive amounts of extras ordered for very aged persons.

30 May. The confinement of the wife of Reuben Miles was used as the reason for application for relief. There had been no order made by the Board but the Relieving Officer had given two gallons of bread per week for four weeks – he said it was given instead of 8/- relief.

James Blagden was also given the same amount for his wife's confinement by the Relieving Officer, again without an order from the Board, and it had not been reported until later. At the same time there was also a complaint that no order had been given for Mary Moore

1878

In October the Board were directed to obtain a certificate signed by a clergyman, churchwarden, Guardian or Relieving Officer, stating that the pauper applying for non-residential relief was living and had no alteration in circumstances. Obviously there had been some cases of fraudulent claims.

4 June. The Guardians received a letter from the Local Government Board enclosing correspondence from a man who had been refused out-relief for himself and wife. The Clerk was directed to inform the Local Government Board that the Guardians did not consider that the case on the whole was a subject for out-relief especially as the paupers involved were dirty in their habits and there was reason to believe that the man earned about 6/- a week.

On 12 February R.C.Glass handed to the Board a letter received from W.Gauntlett, foreman of the Jury at the inquest on Amelia Cummings with a copy of the verdict enclosed. This said she had died from inflammation of the lungs accelerated by an absence of proper food and clothing and that the Jury desired to call the attention of the Guardians to the case in order that the mother of the deceased might receive some out-door relief. The Board directed the Clerk to reply to W.Gauntlett stating the true facts of the case and to ask the editor of the Devizes Advertiser to insert a copy of their reply in the paper as the verdict had been printed in that paper.

Letter addressed to W.B.Gauntlett Esq.

Dear Sir,

In reply to your letter addressed to Relieving Officer Glass, enclosing a copy of the verdict of the jury at the inquest on Amelia Cummings, I am directed by the Board of Guardians of the Devizes Union to bring before you some of the facts relating to the case. It might be sufficient to say that the Guardians are absolutely forbidden by law to grant out-relief to Mrs Cummings, because she has become the mother of a bastard child. Even if this had not been so the Guardians believe that they would have been wrong to contribute towards the maintenance of a household, the disgraceful state of which has for a long time occupied their attention.

Mrs Cummings house was so overcrowded and filthy that, until a number of its inmates had been reduced by the absence of one child, the imprisonment of another for theft, and the death of a third (for whom the mother had not taken the trouble to procure the parish doctor), the Guardians were proceeding to enforce an order they had obtained prohibiting the overcrowding of the house.

Had not the mother been assisted by the alms of well-meaning but mistaken people, she would be living in comparative comfort in the Workhouse, and her children would be well cared for and well educated instead of being left open to the influences of crime, disease and dirt.

I am, dear sir, yours faithfully,

Fredk. M. Lush, Clerk to the Board.

The General Register Office records show that the only Amelia Cummins who had died at the date was a three year old child listed in the Jan/Feb/Mar quarter for 1878.

1881

19 April. It was resolved in cases of people applying for relief who receive assistance from public charities that the amount of such assistance shouldn't be taken into consideration if it did not exceed 1/- a week and if it did exceed that amount it should be estimated at one half.

1882

A poster dated 28 November was signed by Alex Meek, Chairman of Devizes Union, and contained the following information.

The Guardians of the Poor have resolved that in future out-door relief will be allowed only to those persons of good character who can satisfy the Guardians that their destitution has not been caused by their improvidence or intemperance and that whilst at work they have done what they could to make provisions for times of sickness and want of employment. Applicants who are unable to comply with these regulations will, if relieved at all, be required to go into the House with their families.

Outdoor Relief will not be granted (except in cases of sickness or under special circumstances) to the following classes:-

Persons residing out of the Union. Single able-bodied persons. Married women (with or without families) whose husbands have deserted them. Married women (with or without families) whose husbands have been convicted of any offence, and are in prison undergoing the sentence. Persons living in houses which are overcrowded and unfit for human habitation. Persons who are living by themselves and who, by reason of old age or infirmity, are unable to wait upon themselves. Wives and children of soldiers, sailors, militia men in training or the reserve forces to only receive help by a loan. Persons having relatives who are liable and able to maintain them also those living with relatives not legally liable to support them but whose income is fully sufficient to enable them to do so. When in any such cases out-door relief is rendered necessary by reason of temporary illness, it should be given by way of loan. Funeral expenses are not allowed in any case except on condition that the burial is conducted as an ordinary pauper funeral. When estimating the means of any applicant payments from clubs and friendly societies and other pensions should be calculated at one-half the amount.

The Guardians at the same time expressed their earnest hope that all persons residing within the Union would endeavour by thrift and economy to make some provision for themselves instead of relying on the assistance of the Parish and becoming a burden to the ratepayers, all of whom have to contribute towards the amount given in relief, and many of whom are little, if any, better off than those in receipt of relief.

1887
The Board agreed to pay 2/6d per week for Hannah Alford at Miss Smith's Home, she being of weak intellect and unfit for service.

1905
In December Sarah Weston, an inmate previously in the Asylum but now completely recovered, was anxious to find employment and her request for out-door relief for a short time was granted.

Elizabeth Robbins and her 4 children were in receipt of out-relief at 7, Hare & Hounds Court. Mr Drew, one of the Guardians for St John's, reported that on the previous Saturday he visited the home of this pauper. He found only the children in the house, the mother having gone out wooding. Not only was the house in a dirty condition but the children also and he was of the opinion that the family could be much better cared for in the House. A decision was postponed until the next meeting so that the Medical Officer could visit and report back to the Committee. He found the children to be fairly well clad but their clothes were very dirty. The house was exceedingly dirty and neglected. Bedding was disgusting with dirty blankets covered with filth and grease. He felt the children should be removed from such insanitary surroundings as he did not consider it to be a fit place to have charge and control of children. The Committee resolved that relief would continue for 1 week and that an order for admission to the House would be given.

1906

The Board considered a long report about 'feeble minded paupers'. The Guardians gave directions to all the Officers to render every assistance to Dr. Pearce who had been appointed by the Local Government Board to note and classify the mental defectives and the Medical Officers and Relieving Officers were asked to give numbers of mental defectives receiving out-relief.

1908

On the 24 November an application was received from a young woman for relief on behalf of her orphan siblings, their mother having died. They were Dorothy 14, Elizabeth Jane 11 and Henry 9. Their older sister was prepared to become their foster parent. After checking that the sleeping accommodation was satisfactory the Board agreed to give discretionary relief once there was a positive report from both the Medical Officer and the Relieving Officer.

Stratton Sons & Mead Ltd., announced their intention of again making a present of a quarter of a pound of tea to each pauper in receipt of relief in Devizes and Roundway during the Christmas week. Letters were received from Bradford-on-Avon, Westbury and Gloucester Unions regarding extras for out-relief being increased for out-door poor during the winter months. Trowbridge and Melksham were also said to be giving extra and Devizes decided to do the same. Calne, Salisbury and Swindon would give for Christmas week only. Malmesbury declined to give any extra.

1915

Extra relief was to be granted to out-door poor due to increased cost of living because of the war.

1916

It was recorded in the Minutes that a widow's settlement was not accepted for the first year of widowhood as widows were irremovable during that period.

A letter was received from the Birmingham Union about Emily Dixon, a widow of Great Cheverell, asking for a refund of 4/- per week towards her maintenance - non-residential relief was authorised.

George Goddard, late of Chirton, died in Salisbury General Infirmary. There had been no time to communicate with the Relieving Officer therefore Salisbury Union had paid for the funeral expenses of £3.1.0d. He had been admitted from Chirton by order of Dr Stone. As neighbouring Unions always repaid them, Salisbury would be glad if Devizes would do so in this case. After discussion it was agreed that Devizes would pay the funeral expenses.

September. A 41 year old woman and her two children, late of Roundway, were living in Merthyr Tydfil. That Union had granted her out-relief of 10/6d weekly plus 20 per cent War Relief and Devizes was asked if it would accept chargeability without an Order. As she had been on out-relief up to 9 August it was resolved to accept chargeability. It was noted in 28 November Minutes that the family had returned to Devizes from Merthyr.

In November agreement was given for extra relief to be allowed for the out-door poor. This was to be for the Christmas period only. Each adult was to get 2/- and children 1/-.

1927

February. A letter was sent to Calne Union requesting them to accept chargeability for Mary Keel aged 68 and to authorise out-door relief. Calne agreed.

On the 20 September out-relief was authorised for Daisy May Yarnold, who had 3 dependent children, at the rate of 13/- per week for 6 weeks. Her settlement was Kensington and that Union would reimburse the expenditure.

1930

The Minutes show that non-residential relief was still occurring regularly.

8

Problems

The Devizes Union had its share of problems – defects in the building, fallings-out amongst the Guardians, staff and inmates as well as with disgruntled rate payers. Many of the incidents appear quite petty but a few must have caused great embarrassment to the Guardians, such as their refusal to allow lady visitors to the House which got into the national newspapers and was strongly condemned and, of course, a horrific murder in 1881.

The wording of some of the entries in the Minute books, the source of many but not all of the following examples, makes the attitude of the Poor Law Commission, the various Committees and the Guardians towards the paupers and the staff, very evident. For example details of paupers who 'escaped' from the Workhouse – after all it wasn't a prison. Leaving could not have been prevented but re-admission after just a short period could be made difficult and unpleasant.

Staff could be sacked immediately (no question of unfair dismissal then) and were poorly paid for very long hours and in the early days had to live in. The various Committees also had their problems as the Poor Law Commissioners as often as not replied to Guardians requests with an outright 'No'.

Some examples of problems follow.

1837

Richard Box, one of the Elected Board of Guardians, sent a letter to the Poor Law Commissioners querying whether any Guardian was at liberty to be present at a Board meeting and vote on a question in which he was personally involved from a pecuniary point of view. In

short he asks 'Is anyone at liberty to vote money to himself?' Mr Box
goes on

> The Clerk (Tugwell) is a partner in the firm of Salmon, Tugwell and
> Meek (Attorneys) and Mr Salmon is also a Guardian. The firm have
> charged the Union for filling up the bakers' contracts at 10/- and
> 10/6 each time that a contract is entered into, though no order has,
> I believe, ever been given by the Board. When a query was raised the
> invariable practice of the Board had been to ask the person involved
> to leave the room. Mr Salmon would not and said that he would not
> forfeit his rights and privileges as a Guardian. I believe that neither the
> Chairman nor any other Guardian made any observation. The next
> week, in order to settle the question, I proposed that no Guardian,
> nor any other gentleman, should be present whilst any subject is being
> discussed in which he is personally interested. The Vice Chairman
> then proposed an amendment that my proposition be not taken into
> consideration which was almost unanimously carried. This leaves me
> no remedy but an appeal to the honourable Board. The Guardians
> who are in trade think it is not legal for them to supply the Union
> with anything they sell and they do not offer to supply any of the
> contracts which they otherwise would do. Should not the same
> restrictions apply to the professions? Salmon, Tugwell and Meek's bill,
> entered in the ledger for the quarter ending 29 September, was £42
> for contracts and stamps. I think, with many other Guardians who
> have taken an active part in the proceedings of the Board that Messrs
> Salmon & Tugwell's influence is so extensive that they can at times
> obtain a majority on almost any question affecting themselves and
> hence we are compelled to conclude that it will be perfectly useless to
> give time and attention to it. Consequently I am fully persuaded that
> the Devizes Union will not possess those advantages which the new
> Poor Law intended as long as the Clerk to the Union is a lawyer and
> while he is a partner in the most influential office in the county.

The Poor Law Commission replied within a week and said the
matter was being looked into and the very next day sent a letter headed
'Charges for Professional Services' requesting a copy of the accounts

from Salmon, Tugwell and Meek for the last two quarters.

The next month Richard Box got a letter entitled 'For your information herewith a copy of a letter addressed to Mr Tugwell. There is not a copy in the Minutes although there is a copy of a letter signed by Tugwell which states 'No land charges have been made except the cost as stated for the purchase of the land'. Perhaps relevant?

In the same year there appears to have been some conflict between one of the Medical Officers and a local clergyman. The Medical Officer, William Tucker of Market Lavington, was informed by the Poor Law Commissioners 'No clergyman has any authority to interfere in the management of the poor. A proviso followed –it was conceded that the Medical Officer should be grateful to a clergyman for informing him of a fact and ought, under ordinary circumstances, to give the earliest attention to the case pointed out by him. It was emphasised that a clergyman could only suggest but had no power to issue any order'.

7 March. Summonses for non-payment of poor rates had been issued against a large number of poor persons in District 1. They were really unable, through poverty, to pay the same but against whom the Overseers were obliged to obtain summonses, the Magistrates being by law the only persons empowered to excuse them from such payment. It was suggested that an application be brought before T.Estcourt to bring the subject before the Committee of the House of Commons which had been appointed to enquire into the operation of the Poor Law Act. (Very usefully Estcourt was not only Chairman of the Board of Guardians but also a Member of Parliament).

1838
The Visiting Committee recommended that a screen be erected outside the window in the women's ward to prevent the introduction of any spirits or other things through the window.

1839
In September a letter was sent to the Clerk of the Poor Law Commission from the Board.

The previous day, Mr Wilson the Master, complained of the extremely violent conduct of two females named Harriet Alford and Caroline Russ. Alford had been sent to prison and Russ only spared from the same punishment in consequence of her having a disease of the spine and had therefore been punished in the House by a distinguishing dress. All these measures were to no avail and the general conduct of the women continued as bad as ever. The Board, having consulted the surgeon in respect of Russ, ordered the Master to place them in separate rooms for one week and supply them with nothing but bread, making up in that the full weight of allowance in other provisions. Alford, having a child which had been weaned about a month, was allowed to have it with her. The two rooms chosen for the women were the lying-in room (which happened to be vacant) and one of the Receiving rooms. The Board did not consider that the separation they ordered was at all identical with confinement in the lock-up room where straw only is supplied and no light admitted. On the contrary they regarded it as carrying out the discipline of classification, certainly to the extreme point, but that was when all other means had failed and when it was judged absolutely necessary for the peace of the establishment. Such was the state of things at your visit. You then ordered the Master to let the women re-join their usual wards as their confinement was illegal and even with the Master explaining that it was not his own but the expressed order of the Board, you told him that if he preferred their order to that of the Poor Law Commissioners he would lose his place. As you in no way communicated with the Board or any individual connected with it this account, of course, is only what was elicited from the Master when the Board found their order infringed. The Board submits to you that it is absolutely essential that the due authority of the Board should be indicated and also that no Assistant Commissioner has any power to alter the legal classification, especially without any communication from him, and that the power claimed by the Board is altogether necessary for the maintenance of due order.

No apparent reply to this letter is listed in the Minute Book but in late September a letter from Colonel A'Court announced the retirement of Mr Adey as Assistant Poor Law Commissioner. This may or may not be of relevance.

The Committee was asked to report on the relative advantages of Phillips and Willett's Lunatic Asylums. The Board wrote to the Poor Law Commission asking whether Phillips could receive payment for the keep of lunatics who had refused to transfer to Mr Willett, without the express consent of parish overseers and the signatures of two justices. Some parishes had allowed transfer but others had not. This appears to have gone against the decision of the Board dated 1836 when the parish officers were directed that all lunatic paupers be at once given up to Thomas Phillips who was authorised to receive them on agreed terms.

1845

There were problems in enforcing smallpox vaccinations for children due to the prejudice of parents and also because the supply of vaccine from London was of inferior quality.

1861

A decision of the Board led to national coverage in the newspapers. It was proposed by Mr Richard Hill and seconded by Mr Barrey that the application of the Reverend A.Smith for leave for five ladies (all to be named in advance) to visit aged and young paupers at reasonable times and under proper regulations be acceded to. Mr John Harding moved an amendment which was seconded by Mr Fowler that it be NOT acceded to and that no alterations be made in the regulations of visitors attending the House which was carried by a majority of Guardians present. Although there must have been much discussion about the adverse press coverage decisions about the visitors access question did not change for many years illustrated by the fact that in April 1883 the Board also decided to refuse a request from a Miss Edwards to visit four times a year. The reason given was that it would be making a precedent in favour of similar applications.

The Master was directed not to sell vegetables from the Workhouse garden to the gardener. (The vegetables were meant to be used for the inmate's diet and not for the Master or gardener to pocket the proceeds.) They got away with a telling off.

1874

14 April. A letter from W.Carless was received complaining that the child of Arter of the Potterne Road had not been brought for inspection after vaccination. The Clerk was directed to prosecute the father for the default.

In June an enquiry was made about Mrs Perkins who had been offered an affordable home and maintenance at the White Lion. It was ordered that the case be watched and if it was found that the reports of her being ill-treated were true she should be given relief and her case brought before the Board.

1875

One of the Vaccinating Officers was insane and unfit to be personally served his severance. The Clerk was to make sure that this was done in a legal way.

1877

The Relieving Officer informed the Board that a married woman named Cross had died of starvation at Great Cheverell and that until it was too late he had not been informed of her requiring relief. W.Bennet, the Relieving Officer, reported that the husband of the woman who died had absconded. The Board was to enquire into the subject.

A complaint was made that the bread supplied was bad – a loaf was produced but the Board did not think there was a fair cause of complaint. It isn't recorded whether the complaint was made by the staff or by the inmates, neither does it tell whether the Board actually tasted the bread.

The Inspector called to the attention of the Board the large amount of beer consumed in the Workhouse.

1878

23 April. A letter was received from the Local Government Board complaining that a man in the sick bay, Thomas Giddings, had not

been sufficiently attended to. The Guardians were looking into this and also the claim that a boy had not received proper care. The Guardians requested the Clerk to reply that the boy was not in the infirmary at the time of the Inspector's visit because he was then under the care of his mother in another part of the Workhouse and that he had later been removed to the Infirmary and had died there.

1882
A letter was received from the Governor of Devizes prison by which it appeared that the Local Government Board considered that if a prisoner on his discharge was destitute of clothing the Relieving Officer was bound to furnish such clothing as might be necessary to meet the man's immediate needs. The Chairman undertook to write to the Local Government Board and protest against this assertion.

1905
On 5 September the Clerk reported that it appeared from the accounts that several parishes were in arrears with collection and payment of their rates. They were ordered to pay by the 19 September at the latest and were to get a letter to that effect saying that unless they paid at once the Board would take proceedings. The threat obviously did the trick as the next set of accounts show that the payments were made.

1950
In July there were complaints regarding the great difficulty in providing an optician to examine patients for spectacles and this needed to be expedited. This problem continued as in July the Medical Officer again emphasised the need to find an optician interested in providing this service.

1964
For the time of the year the waiting list had never been so long (21 females and 4 males). Dr Varian, in close collaboration with Matron, discussed the mobility and morbidity of each case but failed to find any additional vacancy. The figures for the quarter showed that ten patients had died, fifteen had been discharged and thirty admitted.

There were also ten patients in Devizes Hospital awaiting transfer to St James.

STAFF

1836

A complaint was made against William Maslen, the Master, for leaving the House at a time when the porter had gone out. The Board investigated this and found it to be correct. After being reprimanded it was noted that if he did it again he would be immediately dismissed. The Porter was also reprimanded and told he was on no account to be absent from the House at the same time as the Master.

1838

It had been reported that some of the paupers had been employed by the Master and Matron in carrying letters outside the Workhouse on their own private business. Mrs Cozens was reprimanded and she apologised and promised never again to suffer any pauper being sent out of the House without proper authority. She stated that the paupers would not have been employed in the manner complained of had she been aware that there was any impropriety in her so employing them.

1839/40

In April the Master complained that the Porter, Henry Hazell, had again absented himself from the Workhouse in the night time and asked that he be discharged. A new Porter, Samuel Stiles of Poulshot was appointed in his place.

A letter was sent to the Clerk of the Poor Law Commission from the Guardians because there had been a complaint made to the Board that there was much irregularity in the Workhouse and a great want of cleanliness proceeding from the state of health of Mrs Cozens and the circumstances of the Master and Matron not being husband and wife (Mr Cozens had died in 1838). The Guardians present unanimously agreed that the duties of Master and Matron could not be properly discharged by any persons other than man and wife and that it would be most beneficial to the Union if two persons, being husband and wife, were Master and Matron instead of the Master and Mrs Cozens. Mr Maslen, appeared before the Board and being made acquainted of their opinion and wishes, expressed himself as ready to resign his situation as Master of the Workhouse and straight away tendered his resignation and Mrs Cozens did the same. The Board accepted subject to the approval of the Poor Law Commission. It was suggested that Mrs Cozens could be employed as Supervisor or Head Nurse. This was carried by a majority of 14 to 13. Mrs Cozens asked for time to consider before giving any reply but she later sent a letter declining the appointment. (Probably wisely as it appeared that only half of the Guardians wanted her to stay on). As she had refused the new position she was 'ordered' to leave the House.

1854
The porter was discharged for making a female inmate pregnant.

1861
The schoolmistress was accused of striking a little girl on the shoulder. She confirmed that she had acted in defiance of the Workhouse regulations and she expressed regret at what she had done and promised to do so no more.

1863
The Master reported the schoolteacher, Charles Porter, with having assaulted a little boy aged 10, bruising his face and causing pain. The schoolmaster was called and he did not deny having struck the boy which he excused on a moment of passion. Subsequently he sent in his resignation which was accepted by the Board.

Another report was made about the Industrial Teacher who was accused of slapping two 'weakly' girls and her suspension was requested. She was called in and admitted having hit the girls. After having the relevant part of the rules read to her she expressed regret at having violated them and promised not to re-offend.

1875
There was an Extraordinary General Meeting of the Guardians

re defalcations (dictionary definition is 'mishandling of funds, misappropriation or embezzlement of money') in the accounts of one of the Relieving Officers. The Board proceeded to consider the discovery that had been made. The Officer involved had sent in his resignation which the Board resolved to accept, a new appointment to be made at the same salary as before. Obviously a popular job as upwards of 60 applications for the post were made. William Henry Springford was appointed.

1879

The Board's attention was drawn to the fact that the porter was not efficient in the discharge of his duties. The Master and the Girl's Superintendent gave evidence that he was drunk and incapable on the previous Saturday. He was immediately dismissed.

A man called Benjamin Purnell got the job, chosen by the majority of the Board. Eight months later Purnell resigned and was asking for a reference. It appeared from the Minutes that he was honest, sober and steady but that his health was not strong enough for the duties of a porter. Probably a good job he left then as there was a very lurid Court case in 1889 when he murdered his wife and was hanged at Devizes prison, all reported in the local paper in great detail. His wife had also worked at the House as Children's Superintendent before they were married.

In September Maria Underwood, a pauper in the House, complained that on her first admission she was stripped in the kitchen of the Workhouse and that the gardener, the porter and two boys came into the kitchen at the time. Ragged and dirty clothes had been given her to put on and the Master declined to report her wish to inform the Board of Guardians of her treatment. Somehow the Board got to hear of this and investigated. It appeared that the woman's clothes were changed in the kitchen but behind a screen according to normal practice. The Guardians resolved she had no grounds for complaint except in respect of the Master not supporting her wish that the Board be informed and that in future the Master should enter all cases in which such a wish was expressed in his report book. It was also agreed that in future any pauper, on being admitted, should change their clothes in the Receiving Ward. Unfortunately the Masters Report Book does not appear to have survived to see if he complied with this. In 1878 the Clerk was authorised to destroy all books and papers belonging to the Union more than 10 years old except those which ought to be retained. Perhaps the Master's book suffered this fate.

1881

It appeared that Emma Biffen, an inmate of the Workhouse, was pregnant and that Giles, the Porter, admitted having intercourse with her. Giles was dismissed. The death records show that the baby, Lydia, died aged 16 months.

The new Porter, J.Dunford, also caused trouble by insulting the Master and he had refused to attend the House Committee when requested to do so - he too was dismissed and his wife, who was cook, also had to leave as they had agreed on appointment that it was a dual post.

29 November. The Board expressed sympathy with the Master and Matron for the trouble they had experienced owing to the violent death of Stephen Coleman, an inmate of the Workhouse and their approbation of the courage shown by Richard Hayward in grappling with the man who killed Coleman, whilst the red hot poker was still in his hand. Coleman was aged 77 and from Worton.

A ballad sheet was produced at the time Charles Gerrish was executed at Devizes Prison for Coleman's murder in 1882.

At eight o'clock on Monday morn
Charles Gerrish crossed the river
No more he'll cuss the income tax
Nor grumble at his liver.

A broadsheet was produced at the same time and described how Gerrish was aged 70 and seemed indifferent to his fate. At his trial he had made use of language that shocked all who heard him. He died without a struggle. His crime was never disputed.

There was a follow-on from this event when the Master was in trouble for ignoring the decision of the Board not to take Isabella Masters before Magistrates to get her committed to an asylum. The

Medical Officer had declared her not to be insane and advised that she should be kept in the Workhouse and the Master to treat her as refractory. The Masters reason for his action was that two paupers had informed him that they were in fear of their lives owing to her. Hassall, the Master at that time, was informed that he should not have taken the steps that he did although they thought that the catastrophe which had recently taken place in the House in the violent death of Coleman was some excuse for him.

1908

A 31 year old ex-soldier was appointed as Male Lunatic Attendant and after one month's trial was said to have 'given every satisfaction'. He earned £25 p.a. with rations and uniform. There is further information about him in the chapter on the First World War. Something went wrong here as he was suspended on the 30 December 1922 and dismissal confirmed on 16 January 1923. No details are given in the Guardians' Minute Book why he lost his job but it must have been quite serious as he was refused a reference.

1914

In April the local papers had a headline 'Singular death of a child – Workhouse nurse exonerated'. Francis Herbert D, 1 year and 10 months old, illegitimate son of a domestic servant. The child had left the Workhouse under the care of his mother but was re-admitted in August. He was unwell and died 3 days later. The nurse reported to the Matron that the child was unwell but no doctor saw the child who was never strong having had diphtheria a year ago when he was attended by Dr Waylen in the isolation hospital. The Matron instructed the nurse to take the child to the infirmary 'when the bell rang' (this would indicate that the doctor had arrived).

Dr Waylen was sent for but he was out so the staff gave the child brandy and water bottles to keep him warm. He collapsed and died before the doctor arrived. At the inquest the doctor confirmed that on his morning visit the bell did not ring (he did not ride his motor cycle so the porter might not have heard him).

1916

There was criticism of the Master's actions regarding an admission. The Medical Officer had reported that Ethel Robbins, who had been in labour for two days (according to her statement) was removed to the Workhouse on 28 June in an exhausted condition. She should have been removed earlier if it was necessary to do so as it was unfair to the nurses and staff of the House generally. However, the Committee decided that they approved of the Master's act in admitting this woman. (A mystery here as her name does not appear in the Admissions Register).

1927

23 August. William Stone, the porter, had been off duty for just under 2 weeks suffering from an injury inflicted by a Casual. (A man travelling the county looking for work). Stone received 18/- National Health Benefit and under the terms of his employment the amount of the benefit should be deducted from his salary. It was decided that as he was injured whilst carrying out his duties no deduction was to be made.

ESCAPING FROM THE WORKHOUSE

1836

4 April. Matilda Bowden, Ann Bayley, Elizabeth Nash, all paupers in the House, transgressed the rules. They had also broken out of the Workhouse and got back in during the night by breaking and levering up some iron rails. The Board ordered that Matilda Bowden be kept on bread and water for 4 days, Ann Bayley and Elizabeth Nash for 3 days and until they severally comply with the orders of the Master and Matron and the regulations of the Workhouse.

1837

Betty Burry was to be deprived of her allowance of cheese for one week as a punishment for leaving the Workhouse without permission.

March – An application was made to the Magistrates to get Susan Perrett of Erlestoke punished for running away and taking the Workhouse clothing with her.

24 October. Ordered that a dress different from the usual Workhouse dress be provided and worn by such paupers as misconduct themselves and that Thomas Neal wear it as a punishment for making his escape out of the House.

In December the Master reported the escape of several paupers who had remained out for the night. He was directed to use a particular dress for all paupers guilty of a similar offence.

1838
John Smith of Urchfont absconded with a whole suite of Workhouse clothes. There are many entries for similar offences – in Marlborough Union a man was even accused of absconding with a truss!

1839
Ann Stokes of Urchfont escaped leaving her two children in the Workhouse. A follow up to this shows that the Mayor of Devizes refused to punish her because the Master of the Workhouse was unable to prove the case he alleged against her, that is, unable to prove that she had deserted her children.

DESERTED AND UNSUPPORTED FAMILIES

1837
14 February. Proceedings were to be taken to punish Jacob Gulliver for deserting his wife and children, and leaving them chargeable to St Mary's.

1874
In August Seth Cooksey, a market gardener at Easterton, had deserted his wife and was to be charged 3/6d a week to maintain his 27 year old daughter in the Workhouse.

P.C. Robert Pickett applied for £7, his expenses during two days and one night searching in Bristol and its neighbourhood for James Weston who had deserted his wife.

In September a warrant was issued against George Hutchins of St Mary's for deserting his children. In December Charles Bridewell of

Potterne was required to pay towards the maintenance of his wife.

The above details are just a sample of entries in the Minutes of the Guardians' efforts to obtain payment towards the maintenance of families in the Work House and they would take the culprit to Court if necessary.

INMATES

1836

James Tilley of Potterne was in the Workhouse and the Board was of the opinion that he was an idle, dissolute person and unwilling to work. They decided he should have no cheese. (This punishment seems to have been quite popular with the Board, presumably not so for the paupers).

The Board was informed that two boys had conducted themselves in an improper manner (no details of their behaviour or names given). They were brought before the board and reprimanded.

1837

In January Harry Hutchins had made his escape from the House with a view to leave his family chargeable to the parish of Etchilhampton. The Parish Officers were to take proceedings to apprehend and punish him.

Sarah Hutchins, daughter of Henry (? Harry shown above) escaped from the House taking some portion of Union dress. Application was to be made to the Magistrates to punish her. This may be the same Sarah Hutchins who had an illegitimate child the previous year.

The Overseer of Etchilhampton was ordered to apply to Harry Hutchins to contribute towards the maintenance of his children now in the Workhouse and in the event of his not contributing to apply to the Magistrates to compel and punish him.

1839

The Master complained that William Gardiner had misbehaved by getting out of the Workhouse and he was ordered to be kept in solitary confinement for 23 hours on bread and water. He had previously been punished for misbehaving but the punishment had not resulted in any improvement. His latest misdemeanour was that in January he had 'run away' with Workhouse clothing and therefore had been threatened with prosecution.

1878

The Master reported that Henry Grant had returned from service with Mr Blake at West Lavington, complaining of ill-treatment. The Board examined the case but found no substantial grounds for the complaint.

1905

William and Thomas Ashfield, two pauper inmates, were in trouble as they had 'frequently and without sufficient reason discharged themselves'. In future each of these paupers were required to give 168 hours or 7 days' notice of their discharge as provided for by section 4 of the Poor Law Act 1899.

1908

13 October William Bartlett was given into custody for refusing to work and using threats towards the Master – he was sentenced to 21 days hard labour.

Henry Cross was continually giving in his discharge and going out for a day or two and then returning. He gave considerable trouble and when outside was a nuisance. It was agreed that the regulations stated that 7 days' notice needed to be given before leaving and this should be enforced.

1914

In March Mary Jane Giddings had misbehaved herself in the House and had used abusive language to the annoyance of the other inmates and the staff. On being brought before the Committee she was severely reprimanded and cautioned.

From the above it can be seen that punishment for any misdemeanour by an inmate could vary from a reprimand to reduction of diet, tobacco allowance stopped, confinement within a special room in the Workhouse or the ultimate punishment – sent before a magistrate when a possible prison sentence could follow. Some of the reasons included in the Minutes include bad behaviour, being noisy or dirty, refusing to work, swearing, malingering, being disobedient, removing workhouse property and, of course, running away.

1951
A patient with senile dementia was very attracted to an open fire and on several occasions nearly set fire to herself.

THE BUILDING

1836
On 20 December 132 paupers had been admitted, transferred from the temporary Workhouse in New Park Street. It is not obvious what they might have slept on as the supply of iron bedsteads was discussed because it had been impossible to get them upstairs. Suppliers were asked for quotes for bedsteads requesting that the heads should not be fixed until they got them upstairs. It wasn't until the middle of January before the contract was awarded and shortly after the new, improved beds arrived it is noted that they were not up to specification.

The Medical Officers were not impressed with the privy arrangements – no lights or ventilation, both of which were felt to be essential to prevent stench and disease.

1837
Edward Clack of Bristol had been given the contract for heating with the proviso that work had to be finished by 14 December 1836. However the apparatus for heating did not answer the purpose and the Board decided to buy a thermometer so that they had full details of room temperatures before approaching the architect and the builder again.

Several of the Guardians expressed their dissatisfaction with the new House and wanted liability for this to be considered.

Just to add to their problems the hot water apparatus was not working. The contractor agreed to send a man to sort this out and also to arrange for someone from the Workhouse to be trained in management of the boiler.

By early February at last some of the problems seemed to have been sorted out with the architect attending and agreeing to instruct the contractors and all the rooms now had heating except one on the men's side and they were sufficiently warm.

1838

The privies were out of order in October which led to the Guardians paying 15/- a quarter to keep them in working order. One can imagine the problems this caused with 168 paupers living in the House.

1874

The urban Sanitary Authority wrote to say that keeping of pigs should be discontinued as this was a 'nuisance'. Reply was that it was not the pigs but a large open pit adjoining. The Board decided that they had to provide earth closets (which local firm W.E.Chivers was contracted to install) and that the pit creating the nuisance be done away with. If earth closets were such an improvement it makes you wonder what the previous arrangements had been.

1910

In January the Master drew the attention of the Board to the lack of a lavatory for the Officers' use. He gave the reason for bringing up this matter as the problems experienced by a London Hospital when there was just one W.C. for patients and staff and several of the staff had suffered from sore eyes. Even in St James Hospital days there were complaints from the staff re lack of proper toilet facilities.

1952

Water pressure was so low ablutions could not be carried out in the upper dormitories.

1964

Bathroom facilities were sadly missed on the male first floor. Some toilets existed but needed repainting. The M.O. recommended the construction of a bathroom on the first floor as many patients had difficulty in negotiating the stairs with some barely able to do so. A further note says that sani-chairs were difficult to place in position and this needed to be corrected by moving the toilet to the end wall.

1971

The Christmas period was uneventful except for a fire which broke out in the main kitchen on Christmas morning. Thanks to help from Roundway Hospital dinner proceeded as usual. The fire was subdued by the staff and the Fire Brigade.

9
Vagrants

What are Vagrants? Persons, often in poverty, who wander from place to place without a home or regular employment or income and survive by begging. Casuals were different – they were people looking for employment and travelling from place to place often for seasonal work.

Tramps were a common sight, often bearded and with their possessions in a billycan swinging from a cord around the neck. They were looked upon with great suspicion of stealing hen's eggs and washing from clothes lines. Beards were out of fashion except for sailors so they stuck out like a sore thumb (*Devizes Voices, David Buxton 1996*).

The Vagrancy Act of 1834 had made begging and sleeping rough against the law – punishment could be two weeks hard labour. By the early 1900s opinions were changing and it was acknowledged that some were genuine, such as discharged soldiers and people down on their luck through no fault of their own. This could be caused by sudden emergencies, seasonable lack of available work or the state of the national economy, but the thought was that there were others who did not deserve compassion as they were idle and dissolute.

1837

No tramp or casual was to be refused a bed for the night if they had no money but as far as possible they should be separated from other inmates. Police were paid as Relieving Officers and tramps would have to go to the Police Station to get an order for admission to the Workhouse.

1839

Hickey, a casual pauper was discharged after the Medical Officer reported him fit to travel.

Catherine Couzens, described as a tramper was according to her statement from Ireland. She was received into the House and delivered of a child. Brought before the Board she was told that she would be discharged when her child was fit to travel.

1844

In January the Board of Guardians' received the following directives from the Poor Law Commissioners

> If casual paupers are admitted for a nights lodging and food at any time before it is dark they are immediately to be set to work to 'pick okum' (this consisted of old ropes). The unravelled product was sent to the docks to caulk ships. They were then to be to be furnished with a supper according to the dietary of the house then sent to bed. If they came in too late in the evening for work they were to fare the same but without any work. When the house bell for rising in the morning was rung they were to be placed in a room set apart for the purpose and to each able-bodied pauper was to be given one third of a day's work as performed by the able-bodied inmates of the establishment and only when they had completed the work were they to have breakfast. If they refused to work they were to be detained for four hours after the hour of rising and discharged without breakfast.

Regard was to be had in each case to the circumstance of the pauper such as a mother with small children and persons who were forced to seek the provisions of the workhouse (not being regular tramps) or the very aged, and in these cases the work was to be forgone or lessened as seemed expedient or necessary.

After 1929 the Medical Officer was required to examine casual and vagrant inmates on admission but sometimes this was changed to only cover those who might, for a medical reason, be unfit to work. The Guardians had informed the Poor Law Commissioners that they had already adopted the above and they had not made any variations in the course of proceeding having found the regulations worked very well.

Vagrants had previously received little sympathy until after 1837 when they were allowed to receive shelter and a meal in return for work. In Devizes this involved cutting up old railway sleepers for firewood for men and scrubbing floors, cleaning, working in the laundry or kitchen, for the women. The Minutes do mention that a bone crusher had been bought but there is no record that this work was actually carried out in Devizes. Bone crushing was, of course, stopped everywhere after the Andover scandal came to light as described in the Incidental's chapter. They also did some stone breaking in Devizes as in 1874 the Surveyor of the Devizes Sanitary Committee offered to pay 8/6d a ton for black rock gravel available from the Workhouse. The cutting up of old sleepers had continued until much later and the Minutes record that in 1905 the Guardians arranged for a cheque to be sent to the Great Western Railway for old sleepers which could be converted into firewood.

Because of increased demand for relief the regulations were tightened to make the work and accommodation as disagreeable as possible. Accommodation was to be in a separate, unheated ward, they had to have a bath on arrival, no smoking or gambling allowed and both men and women were to be locked in at night, sometimes without any bedding. The Board's power to enforce these regulations didn't work very well as tramps were often not in a hurry to get away although those genuinely seeking work needed to leave immediately after breakfast.

After 1843 the authorities gave permission for vagrants to be searched before admission (this was hugely resented) to make sure they were actually destitute and had no money or valuables and also no tobacco but, more reasonably, to make sure they had no weapons such as knives. The hedge adjoining Devizes Workhouse is rumoured to have been the tramps 'bank' where they hid any possessions – I have never heard of anything being found there despite some searches. As late as 1915 directives were received by the Board that casual poor and destitute wayfarers, admitted by the police or Workhouse Master, were to have any money taken away from them, not to be returned when they left, so maybe the rumours of a 'Bank' in Sedgefield gardens has some basis!

The trade depression in the 'Hungry Forties' led to a huge increase in people requiring relief but the Poor Law Board did not take this into account and claimed the regular provision of food and lodging at the public expense was leading to abuse of relief.

In some Unions deliberate tearing up of their clothes by vagrants took place, this meant they got 'new' clothes. This was a serious offence and the perpetrator could go to prison. It was also suggested that this was done to avoid the workhouse for what might be better conditions in prison. There is no evidence that this took place in Devizes.

1846

Some statistics for Vagrants and Tramps admitted to the Workhouse during one week just before Christmas.

Males.
December
13   1 in 16-60 age group.
17   2 in under 16 and 5 in 16-60 age group.
18   2 in 16-60 age group.
19   1 under 16 and 7 in 16-60 age group.
Only 2 in the 16-60 age group were females.

In the previous year the figures for the same week were 14 males and 5 females.

The Minutes regularly give details of the number of vagrants at any one time and from these it is easy to see how the numbers changed from year to year and also how the monthly changes could indicate availability of work, bad weather and national events (such as war) although there are occasional drops or rises not immediately understandable.

1858

The attitude of ratepayers to tramps is illustrated by an article in the *Devizes Advertiser*. Entitled 'Beggars' it states 'The public are against several able-bodied men belonging to the parish of Urchfont who are begging about this town under the plea that they are unable to obtain employment in their parish during the winter months, after having worked all the summer months for Mr Butler. This story is altogether untrue. They make a very plausible and presentable tale, every word of which is false. Like the greater proportion of street beggars they are utterly worthless characters, unable to work as other do and equally unwilling in their distress to go to the Union Workhouse which is the proper refuge for the destitute'.

1861

The Casual Act tightened up the regulations. Casuals were not to be allowed to leave until 11.00 a.m. on day after arrival and only after completing their allotted task. The regulations dictated that if he or she came back after 1 month to have 1 day's hard labour and be held until 11.a.m. on the third day.

1879

In May the vagrant numbers had risen considerably compared to the number for the same period the previous year (from 86 to 146).

1881

17 May. The report of the Committee on Vagrancy adopted by the Quarter Sessions was laid before the Devizes Board. They agreed to all the recommendations except for the one isolating vagrants in separate cells. It was considered that the suggestion that vagrants should be detained during Sundays was most desirable and the Board applied to the Local Government Board for authority to make such detention.
Confirmation was received that they might detain vagrants who entered the Work House on Saturday nights over Sunday until the performance on Monday morning of their task of work. The House Committee was asked to advise the Board what arrangements could be made to accomplish this and decided that the Relieving Ward could be used for the detention of male vagrants during Sundays and a proper person should be found to look after them. The female vagrants sleeping ward would be sufficient for the accommodation of the very

few female vagrants who were likely to be in the house on Sundays. The Board then authorised the Master to carry out these arrangements. 18 October. A Circular was read from the Clerk of the Peace confirming that arrangements had been made for the issue of tickets or papers to vagrants for providing them with midday relief at Beckhampton, Chippenham, Lyneham, Marlborough, Melksham, Pewsey, Trowbridge, Upavon, Warminster and West Lavington.

1882

The regulations were tightened up even more but at a later date casuals could leave earlier if they were trying to get work.

In January Mr Thomas Tyler, the new Inspector of Police at Devizes, was appointed as Relieving Officer for Vagrants at a salary of £10 p.a. The appointment was to expire on his ceasing to be an Inspector at Devizes.

The present Receiving Room was to be used as a day-room for vagrants and the lumber and carpenter's room was to be divided and one part used as a Receiving Room.

1885

A circular from the Chief Constables Office in Devizes was addressed to the inhabitants of the County of Wilts.

There is now in force a system for the relief of destitute wayfarers throughout the County of Wilts. A ticket received by the wayfarer from the Assistant Relieving Officer for the Union where he is passing the night ensures him a midday meal of bread sufficient to carry him on to the Union where he intends sleeping that night. The public are therefore earnestly WARNED against giving to strange beggars, as by so doing they encourage idle vagabond habits which causes an increased expenditure from the rates. Beggars should be referred to the nearest Constable. Male and female destitute persons passing through the County are provided for by night at the Union Workhouse and by day with bread administered under the direction of the Police at certain relief stations.

This Way Ticket was intended almost as a bribe to make sure they moved on to an intended destination but it was misused and consequently abandoned.

Vagrant/Casuals deaths in Devizes Union Workhouse 1866 – 1902

Jemima Chivers aged 51, died 27/1/1890
William Halligham aged 46, died 31/8/1897
Maud Rampton aged 2, died 21/2/1889
William.Robinson aged 64, died 22/1/1887
William Rose aged 47, died 11/10/1889
George Smith aged 40, died 10/8/1891

All the burials took place in Devizes Cemetery.

Census returns showing names of vagrants

The parish of Settlement gives an indication of how far and wide some of these men travelled.

1841 – No vagrants noted

1851
William French aged 46, unmarried, shoesmith Hertfordshire
Daniel Talbot aged 72, Kerry, Ireland

1861
George Adams aged 56, widower, excavator, Dorset,Broad Windsor
John Stone aged 40   No details listed.

1871
George Cook aged 30 Kent
– Edwards aged 53 Northumberland
Edwin Andrew aged 30 Berkshire
William Collins aged 45 Axminster, Devon

1881
William Ruskin aged 63 Northampton
William Hidder(?) aged 35 Bath
Thomas Dark aged 39 London
James Neville (?) aged 23 Reading

1891
George Hedges aged 39 Maidstone
John O'Brian aged 37 Dublin

1901
George Young aged 28 Cirencester
William King aged 65 Wimbourne
Thomas Cox aged 21 Northampton

1911
None noted as in the Workhouse the night of the census.

Examples of numbers of vagrants relieved

Increase or decrease of numbers over corresponding date the previous year.

23 Dec 1873	22 (increase of 11)
3 Mar 1874	30 (increase of 14)
14 April 1874	16 (decrease of 7)
28 April 1874	34 (increase of 7)
30 May 1874	16 (increase of 3)
23 June 1874	35 (increase of 34)
7 July 1874	13 (no change)
21 July 1874	21 (increase of 2)
4 Aug 1874	9 (decrease of 17)
18 Aug 1874	26 (increase of 5)
7 Sept 1874	18 (decrease of 7)
15 Sept 1874	29 (increase of 12)
29 Sept 1874	21 (increase of 13)

13 Oct 1874	29 (increase of 14)
27 Oct 1874	47 (increase of 17)
10 Nov 1874	56 (increase of 32)
24 Nov 1874	20 (increase of 6)
8 Dec 1874	26 (increase of 6)
22 Dec 1874	20 (decrease of 2)
5 Jan 1875	11 (increase of 1)
19 Jan 1875	16 (decrease of 1)
1 Jan 1878	77 (increase of 53)
15 Jan 1878	95 (increase of 61)

In 1915 the numbers were down from the previous year. This decrease occurred all over the country at the start of the First World War, some Unions even closed their casual wards but numbers shot up after the end of the war when there was a period of high unemployment.

28 Nov 1916	51 (decrease of 15)
27 Dec 1916	28 (decrease of 33)
27 Nov 1917	14 (decrease of 11)
16 Nov 1926	408 (increase of 124)
14 Dec 1926	380 (increase of 55)
8 Feb 1927	428 (increase of 38)

1874
23 June. The Local Government Board requested that the vagrants ward be provided with a bath and a bell.

1882
4 April. A circular was read from the Local Government Board regarding vagrants spreading infectious diseases, particularly smallpox. The clerk was directed to draw this to the attention of the Master and the Relieving Officer for vagrants.

1889
On 5 December the *Wiltshire Gazette* reported that a Casual at Trowbridge Union House named John Smith, refused to do his

allotted task at the Workhouse. He was given into custody, admitted the charge and said he wished to get to Devizes to see a doctor. He was therefore sent to Devizes for 10 days.

1908

On the 14 August Chippenham Union asked if the Board were adopting the recommendation which had been arrived at during the meeting of delegates at Trowbridge on 13 May.

Chippenham Board were anxious to give gruel instead of water for breakfast. Devizes Union Board felt that unless other Workhouses in the County did the same the Chippenham tramp wards would be inundated with vagrants.

It was agreed that a uniform diet for vagrants was important. The Board explained that for some years past they had issued gruel for breakfast and insofar as accommodation would permit the recommendations of the conference were being carried out. Also the Guardians of this Union were not only strongly of opinion that there should be uniformity in the treatment of vagrants in this County and that it would be an excellent thing were the Unions in the adjoining counties prevailed on to adopt similar measures.

In October the House Committee again considered the question of supplying gruel for tramps. It was felt that a too generous distribution had been given to undeserving casuals and recommended that in future the Master use his discretion in supplying gruel only to the deserving.

27 October. Vagrants in house 96, increase of 39 from same period the previous year.

1909

Owing to a large increase in the number of vagrants due to the Depression the Board was asked to give an increased amount towards the cost of providing mid-day relief. They agreed to increase this from £3.5.0d to £4 per annum. In June 1910 this rise in numbers had continued with an increase of 51 vagrants relieved over the same period last year.

1910

There was protracted discussion by the Guardians about a suggested clause in the Local Government Board's Order of 23 September. The following details were recorded in the Minutes.

This Order contemplates that the mid-day meal shall, if practical, be given at a way- station in pursuance of an agreement with a Vagrancy Committee. The dietary table provided that the mid-day meal should consist of set amounts of bread and cheese for men, with less amounts of these for women and children. In the case of children under 8 years, then half a pint of milk with the addition for those under 3 years of half an ounce of sugar should be allowed. Because of the difficulty of storing milk at the way- station then the milk should be given in a bottle by the Workhouse where the casual pauper had passed the previous night. The simplest way would be for a ticket to be given to each vagrant for relief at the way-station on his road.

No doubt the additional cheese would greatly increase the cost but it was hoped that the ampler sustenance would prevent the public from giving alms to strange beggars which had been the greatest encouragement to vagrancy.

The Board, when asked for their opinion, pointed out that this could only work if supported by every Union in the Country and unanimously resolved that the above suggestion of the County Vagrancy Committee be approved.

1914

In the case of a vagrant admitted to the workhouse who died there the words 'admitted as a vagrant' were to be inserted in the death records. After 1914 the wording was changed slightly to read 'where a person has been admitted from a place other than his usual place of abode this should also be stated if known'. In the official death ledgers there are entries in the early registers of 'Vagrants' but none noted between 1908 and 1914 or in a second book for dates covering 1914 to 1939. In March a proposal came from Warminster Union that an increased diet for vagrants to include 8oz of bread and cheese as their mid-day meal should be refused.

This was followed later in the month by a letter from the Chairman of the Wilts County Vagrancy Committee stating 'hitherto mid-day relief to tramps had consisted of 8 oz of bread only and that in neighbouring counties a ration of cheese was also allowed'. On consideration of the cost at the last Vagrancy Committee it was estimated that it would involve more than double the cost of relief. The Committee felt it was not in their power to authorise that expenditure without increased contributions, such contributions being based on 2d per £100 of rateable value of each Union and in the case of Devizes would amount to £7.10.00. It was pointed out that for a man or woman making a fair day's march between Unions 8oz of bread alone was very bare subsistence and hardly enough to assure the public that all bona fide wayfarers could obtain sufficient food to carry them through the day. This was a most important matter for consideration as vagrancy could never be reduced to a minimum except by inducing the public to withhold alms from strange beggars. Another consideration was that the county should come into line as far as possible with neighbouring counties in the relief given so as to have as near as may be uniformity of treatment. On the above grounds it was asked for favourable consideration by the Board and if it would be willing to augment the annual contribution named.

It was agreed by the Board to increase the amount of annual grant from £4 to £7.10.00

1915

9 January. A letter from Warminster Union described the discharge of two casuals from the wards of the Devizes Workhouse on a Sunday. The Master reported that as a rule casuals were not discharged on Sundays but the limited accommodation made it necessary to do so occasionally. On Sunday 24 January, owing to the extra number of admissions, they were obliged to discharge two men. The Clerk was to send a letter to Warminster to explain the exceptional circumstances.

1917

27 November. A letter from the Chairman of the County Vagrancy

Committee was received pointing out that it was very desirable that casuals were not discharged on Sundays and hoping it be adopted throughout the County. The Board Resolved to reply that it was not their practice to discharge Casuals from the Workhouse on Sundays and then only in cases of emergency.

1918

April. The Master asked for the Board's instructions in regard to vagrants coming into casual wards with food in their possession. It was resolved that the Master be authorised to use his discretion as to whether, on their discharge, vagrants were to be provided with a meal.

1919

24 November a letter was received from Ministry of Health on vagrancy urging that ex-servicemen should communicate with the local office of the Ministry of Labour and register there.

1921

27 September. The Board reported to the Minister of Health and Wilts Vagrancy Committee the serious increase in the number of Casuals applying for admission due to the casual wards of neighbouring Unions being closed. Devizes Poor Law Institution was not able to meet the needs of all cases.

1924

The Board of Guardians asked for advice on how to deal with the strong increase in the number of Casuals over the last 12 months. This increase appeared to be accounted for by the large number of young men who had never made any serious attempt to obtain work although they were able-bodied. They relied on being maintained either by unemployment benefits or by the Guardians.

1925

Casual Poor (Relief Order). A circular from the Ministry of Health directed that okum picking was to be omitted from the tasks which Guardians could impose upon Casuals.

1926

On the 21 September the Master was instructed to obtain tea and cheese for Casuals, these to be of a cheaper quality than that supplied to the inmates.

1927

8 February. The Master reported an unusual number of admissions to the Casual wards. Owing to overcrowding he had been obliged to allow some of the vagrants to go before completing their stipulated time of detention. The Committee was impressed with the urgency of the Casuals problem and queried the need for more accommodation.

(In November 1926 the number of 'Casual' admissions was 408, which was an increase of 124 over the same period for the previous year).

On the 3 May there was discussion about tramps suffering from contagious diseases. There were no powers to detain and send them for treatment so permission was to be sought.

1928

The Minutes of 18 September showed a proposal for a new Casual Ward. A letter from the Ministry of Health Inspector stated that if the number of casuals could be kept down within existing limits by strict administration it might be possible to avoid expensive additions to the Casual wards for the time being. The Inspector had checked the accommodation at Devizes again and was of the opinion that a drying room ought to be provided, possibly near the boiler room with some other minor changes of use of various spaces. The House Committee were to consider these proposals.

1929

In January the Committee expressed concern about the number of children accompanying vagrants on the roads and wondered if anything could be done to prevent this.

It appeared that numbers had been cut down as on 5 February the number of vagrants relieved was 180 compared with the previous year's figure of 519.

1931

The Public Assistance (Casual Poor) Order instigated less harsh regulations and better diet and accommodation.

At this date the following tramps and casuals are listed. It is noticeable that they all stayed for a minimum of 3 days up to a maximum of 19 days. Casuals are normally thought of as moving on after one or two nights stay and then leaving but this does not seem to have happened in Devizes.

	Admitted	Discharged
Frank Cox, 47, St James	1/3/31	16/3/31
Frederick Tongue, 66, St James	2/3/31	13/3/31
Charles Driscoll, 69, St James. Fireman	8/6/31	11/6/31
John Carter, 19, St James, Labourer	8/6/31	25/6/31
(His mother of 84, London Road, Plaistow, London E14).		
Frederick Rogers, 31, St James, Labourer	10/6/31	29/6/31
John Mortimer, 78, St James, Labourer	30/6/31	10/7/31
Richard Westwood, 44, St James, Labourer	10/7/31	27/7/31
Leonard Cornill, 38, St James, Labourer	24/8/31	28/8/31
Henry Jefferies, 61, St James, Labourer	26/8/31	1/9/31
Thomas Warren, 52, St James, Labourer	27/8/31	12/9/31

1956

In early January some male patients were difficult to handle. One was a vagrant Irishman who caused much disturbance to other patients and the assistance of the police had to be obtained. There are no more entries after this date pertaining to vagrants in the M.Os reports.

10
Wartime and Aftermath

1914

All over the country expenditure on Institutions was being cut. Fortunately the number of admissions had dropped at the beginning of the 1st World War– one reason was that women could find work in factories (for example munitions) and they were also able to claim relief from the National Relief Fund. Also some vagrants were able to take civilian jobs previously filled by men who had joined the services or even joined-up themselves.

27 December. A circular letter from the Local Government Board was sent to all Unions drawing attention to what they described as 'disqualified relief'. This affected the families of men employed on any naval or military service. Instead of help from the Union assistance was available to wives and other relatives of soldiers and sailors from the National Relief Fund. The Guardians were required to provide costs and directed that all entries in the records indicating Poor Law Relief should be erased.

The Soldiers and Sailors Help Society wrote enquiring whether the Board had or were likely to have any openings for attendants suitable for discharged soldiers or sailors. The answer was that there were none at present but sympathetic consideration would be given if any openings occurred.

Measures were to be set up to consider the needs and the distribution of relief caused by the war with the Commissioners responsible for the co-ordination of all relief agencies in the locality both official and voluntary in the event of distress becoming acute. However the Guardians were to continue to deal with all persons who had been in the habit of relying on Poor Law Relief but they should not receive help from the Commissioners and were to be discouraged from applying for such assistance.

At the same time there was to be close co-operation between the Commission and Poor Law Authority Officers especially concerning employees serving as reservists. One of the Devizes staff had left to join the Wiltshire Regiment as a Reservist and it was decided that he was not to be paid but it would be left to the Chairman to call a special meeting to decide if his salary should continue to be paid.

1915

12 January. A circular was received from the Local Government Board regarding British born wives and children of interned aliens and relief of other destitute aliens. The Minutes note that no action needed to be taken by the Guardians as there were none in the Devizes Union area. Wives and widows of soldiers were to be entitled to financial help from the National Relief Fund.

Some Union employees were serving in naval and military forces. The National Poor Law Officers Association had under consideration the effect of the Superannuation Act 1896 upon Poor Law Officers who were serving for the period of the war. It was resolved that posts should be kept open until their return from service and that such service should count for superannuation. If disabled the superannuation allowance should be calculated on the salary and allowances that would otherwise have been received.

In March avoidance of all new work was recommended by the Local Government Board except for pressing necessity. This proposal was put to the Guardians, the reasons given being the unsettled state of the country owing to the war, the increased cost of building materials and scarcity of labour. The Board therefore decided there was no urgent necessity for the provision of a children's home, this being an inopportune time for proceeding with the matter and the Local Government Board should to be asked to consent to a postponement of the whole question until after the close of the war. This was carried with one dissension from the Reverend J. Kingsland. Investigations about a possible children's home at Jump Farm, Devizes, were therefore discontinued. The war ended all sorts of developments not just in

Devizes but all over the country with what were considered to be non-essential services stopped or postponed.

1916

March. Insurance was taken out against Zeppelin raids to protect against damage to the House and premises. This was done at a premium of £8.9.0d p.a.

A circular letter from the Local Government Board gave details of Army Separation Allowances which was to be circulated to Relieving Officers and the Master.

In March Herbert Acutt resumed his duties in the Infirmary after having done his duty with the Colours at the Front. He had been invalided out from the Army but was fortunately able to take up his old position in the Home. David Robbins who had filled Acutt's position during his absence was now released but the Committee recommended that he be employed in the garden. It was explained that for some months, owing to the revision of duties necessary to carry on the work in the House during difficult times, that there had been no regular overseer of the garden work and that in the circumstances it seemed appropriate to offer Robbins the job.

In April there were 3 army pensioners in the House and it had previously been decided that they could keep 8d a week from their pensions. Agreement was reached that this should be increased as follows:-

John Weeks aged 76 to 1/-, James Goddard aged 75 and Robert Orchard aged 66, both to 1/6d.

Also in April Relieving Officer Talbot was concerned whether he was due to be called up and asked if it was it likely that an appeal would be made for a Certificate of Exemption by the Board. The Committee recommended that he submit himself for examination before the Medical Board then sitting at the Devizes Barracks. By June Talbot had received formal notice to join the Colours of the Wiltshire Regiment but had been granted a short extension by the recruiting officer so that he could present his books and accounts to the Board. Mr Glass, his predecessor, had expressed his willingness to carry out the work in his absence. The Clerk had also been informed that Mr

Mitchell, Relieving Officer of District 1, was prepared to take over. The Finance Committee interviewed the two men and they chose Mitchell. He was to be paid £25 p.a. as well as extra fees as Registrar of Births and Deaths, Vaccination Officer and Collector of Rates.

July. The tailor, Sidney Hartnell, a married man with one child, had been called up and had joined the Colours. His wife would get the Separation Allowance of 12/6d and 5/- per week for the child with Hartnell receiving pay of 3/6d per week. The Committee recommended that the allowance be increased by the Board by 5/6d so as to make Hartnell's pay remain the same as what he had been receiving from the Board. Later, however, the increase was turned down as 'having regard to his prospective income it was felt there would be no hardship'. The Soldiers Separation Allowance had been increased in March 1916 and included not only the wife and children of married men but also dependants of unmarried men and widowers. A special claim form had to be filled in at the Recruiting Office and submitted less than one month from the joining up date.

August. The Committee took into account the great increase in work which had fallen upon the Master and Matron during the past 12 months owing to the reduced staff. It was resolved to give them a gratuity of £10 jointly in recognition of their extra services.

Also in August Acutt had again been called up and the Chairman and Master were empowered to offer temporary employment as Imbecile Attendant to Sidney Lacey Crees, aged 23, late Seaforth Highlanders, who had served in the Expeditionary Force in France and was wounded in the foot.

October. The windows in the Chapel were to be darkened to comply with lighting restrictions. This would mean that the time of evening services, which had been put back one hour, could be held at a more convenient time.

The subject of War Bonuses to non-residential staff was discussed. Some members of staff had applied for the Bonus pointing out that this was being paid elsewhere due to the increased cost of living. It was agreed that the male staff should receive 3/- per week and female staff 2/- per week for the period of the war. Those named to receive the extra money were

David Rolfe, engineer up to 30/- per week. David Robbins, Labour Master and W.J.Lovelock Attendant in Infirmary with S.L.Crees, Temporary Imbecile Attendant, all up to 28/- and Clara Elliot (job not specified) up to 14/- per week.

1918

25 April. An Emergency General Meeting was called to discuss a letter from Lord Roundway. Beds and accommodation had to be provided for 18,000 soldiers invalided out of the army and of those Wiltshire would have to provide for 145. If possible the number of beds in any one place should be 30 or more with the Pensions Minister undertaking to provide the full cost of equipment and maintenance. Private houses could not accommodate 30 therefore Lord Roundway had visited the Union House. He had found that the staircases to some of the wards would not be suitable for men who might be badly crippled. The Guardians were asked if they would 'surrender' the infirmary. After consulting the Medical Officer it was realised there would be objections but the claims of 'our gallant soldiers' were very great. After full discussion it was agreed to accommodate 30 wounded soldiers with the proviso that suitable empty houses should be commandeered before any unnecessary disturbance of the Institution happened. A sub-committee was to be set up to administer these arrangements.

Some men, unable to work because of war injuries, became vagrants and the Workhouse became their last resort for relief and because of this the Board was required to notify the War Pensions Committee of any such admissions to the Workhouse.

In August advice was given to the Board that the Mercantile Marines could be of advantage to boys of good conduct who could train both for the Royal Navy and the mercantile services. Particular attention was given to the training offered on the Exmouth, the property of the Metropolitan Asylum Board, to boys with slightly defective vision, if of presentable appearance, for training as stewards, buglers etc., and for strong lads of 16 for training as stokers and trimmers. The circular urged the Guardians to take energetic action at the present crisis.

The Armistice 11 November. The Guardians recorded 'the proud relief, solemn joy and thankfulness to the Almighty God for the victorious ending of the tremendous strife. Its gratitude to the navy, army and air force, to the daughter nations of the Empire and to India for the amazing valour and undoubted self-sacrifice'

1919

8 July. Peace Celebrations. The Local Government Board sent a circular enabling Guardians to make modifications to the regulations for discipline and diet of inmates of the Workhouse and also providing reasonable additions for the outdoor poor in the week of public celebrations. It was unanimously resolved that all adults in receipt of out-door relief should have an extra allowance of 2/6d and all children 1/6d, this to include children boarded out for the week and including Peace Day 19 July. The Master was to be left to make such arrangements as he felt suitable. It was agreed that the inmates should be provided for on a reasonably liberal scale and share with the rest of the community the fullest pleasure of the occasion.

On 5 August it was reported to the Board that the inmates had spent a very pleasant day and wished to thank the Board for providing them with extra fare. As another concession during the afternoon the inmates were allowed out to visit their friends and visitors were also allowed into the house.

October. Letter from the Wilts War Pensions Committee – owing to the railway strike it was possible that it would be necessary for motor transport to be used in connection with sending men to hospitals and hoping the Board would assist so that men requiring treatment could have their cases dealt with as soon as possible.

On 21 January the Chairman reported that he had gone carefully into the question of War Bonuses for the Master and Matron and was of the opinion that the Board could only grant to them one third to one half of the amount granted to the non-residential officers. The Boards' final decision was to make a payment of £7.3.9d to W.Fear and £5 to the Matron, Mrs M.Fear.

1920s

In the inter-war period the largest number of people in Institutions was the elderly and unmarried mothers. With the widespread unemployment after the First World War this caused both financial and overcrowding problems in many Unions. Some injured military personnel had nowhere else to get help other than the House and vagrancy increased, partly due to discharged soldiers looking for employment, and the problem was exacerbated by the fact that many casual wards had been closed during the war.

11
St James Hospital

The Union workhouse became the Poor Law Institution in 1913 but it was the Local Government Act of 1929 that finally ended the Victorian Poor Law and the name was changed again to Public Assistance Institution. However, the Devizes Area Board of Guardians Committee was still in existence in 1939. After the 1948 National Assistance Act the Mid-Wilts Hospital Management Committee was formed and St James Hospital came into being, specialising in geriatrics. The hospital closed in late September 1990. Various archives have been deposited at the Wiltshire & Swindon History Centre and details regarding St James can mainly be found in the Area Health Authority records, although the details of patients are closed for 100 years. Despite this, the reports of the Medical Officer (Dr. Varian)

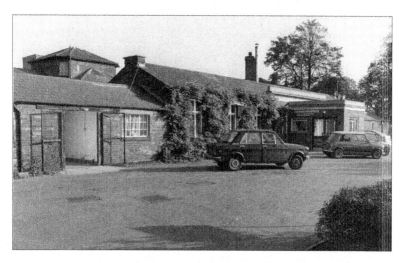

Frontage of St James Hospital shortly before closing

are not closed and give a wide picture of life and conditions in St James Hospital. These indicate not only his medical knowledge but also his and the staffs' concern for the well-being of the patients, no improvement being too small not to be instigated although they understood that large improvements would probably be postponed or even abandoned by the Authority mainly for monetary reasons.

The items which follow come from the Medical Officer's quarterly 'Reports to the Management Committee' covering the period 1947 to 1973 (other entries from this are included in the Vagrants, Health and Building chapters) and extracts are also included from the Visitor's Book, Board of Control Reports and John Willett's publication *Hospital Diary*.

The first entry in the Medical Officer's reports starts at 18 October 1947 when Dr Varian notes that he has loaned an instrument steriliser and ordered certain surgical instruments.

Inmates of the hospital were not just the elderly sick but also children and those categorised as Mental Defectives. In November a child had been admitted on an Order through the NSPCC. In December another patient was admitted via the police with loss of memory. There are notes about a child who had been referred to the Assize Court before being transferred to a children's home. The child was fit but had bruising of her left arm and forearm which may have been caused by a fall. Her young half-sister was in St James Hospital at the parent's request.

The report for the half-year ending 31 December 1947 stated that the feeding of patients was excellent, care of wards good, and the service of a Chiropodist of great help. The beds in the Infirmary were utilised to capacity and the nursing staff gave great attention and care to the patients with full co-operation from both admin and nursing staff.

A nice touch – Dr Varian tells of Christmas Day festivities which he felt were a great success. He attended on Christmas Day and assisted in serving dinners. Being a qualified surgeon one supposes he carved the meat.

In February 1948 an interesting case. A seriously ill woman of 82 was admitted in a dying condition suffering from pernicious anaemia. Her condition became satisfactory after a blood transfusion. March was an exceptionally busy one, beds in the infirmary filled as soon as empty and deaths almost entirely confined to those cases admitted in a dying condition.

March 1949 – Infirmary very crowded and beds difficult to find for urgent cases. Shortage of beds continues to be noted in Dr Varian's reports throughout the years and his worry that patients who should be in St James were bed blocking in Devizes Hospital.

Occupational Therapy had been started with a part-time therapist but had failed to make an impression on the male side. Many senile men were lethargic and set in their habits and it was difficult to arouse their interest. A later entry shows that the patient's attitudes had improved and it was proving a success and had been declared to be of great benefit.

January 1953 – All patients admitted to the Infirmary, if their condition permitted, to have a general bath and hair-wash. In this connection it sometimes being difficult to dry the women's hair, it was recommended that an electric hair-dryer be supplied.

Period ended 8 July 1955. Admissions were average with a tendency to ease off during June. A number of cases remained in hospital having arrived from other areas during a period of bed shortage elsewhere. Efforts were being made to transfer these patients to their proper area but it was understood that transfers did not occur until the waiting list of urgent cases had been cleared. Ward work had proceeded uneventfully although staff shortages had occurred from time to time, but these were of a temporary nature.

October 1955 – Admissions were steady with few empty beds and with a very small waiting list. The M.O. considered that the type of bath in use throughout the hospital was of a very obsolete pattern being much too deep to allow easy handling of patients. His advice was that these baths should be replaced by a modern type when funds became available.

It had been very gratifying to the Matron, Nursing, Medical and Admin staff to receive so many letters of appreciation from patients and patients' relatives. It was felt that the reputation of the hospital was being speedily enhanced.

January 1956. Christmas festivities had come and gone and were enjoyed by staff and patients alike. Fortunately few of the latter were seriously ill and a pleasant and relaxed atmosphere was maintained. The present 'flu epidemic had so far passed St James by and the illnesses on the ward were mainly those usual for the patients' age group.

By April 1958 there was still a small waiting list but this was negligible compared with other regions. However, full bed capacity was seldom in use due to the difficult access to the upper wards and the disability of the average patient.

An entry in October the same year illustrates the Medical Officer's concern in matters not strictly medical. He says 'Unable to use grounds and out-door facilities due to wet and unreliable weather. I am dissatisfied with the condition of the courtyard between the male block and kitchen and admin block. The surface has broken up and the wet weather has encouraged the growth of weeds and general untidiness. Resurfacing recommended when funds available'. He notes that one year later nothing had been done and the same problem still existed. A note is again made in July 1961 'Untidy, weed infested and paper strewn areas remain as before − reported over the last 2 years to no effect'.

Another complaint is made in 1959 that there was inadequate lavatory accommodation mainly in the female ambulatory wards. Nocturnal frequency was a problem and the practice of having to queue at night considered altogether unsatisfactory.

October 1972. Because of work being carried out on the wards all admissions, except urgent cases, had been suspended. Full admissions from the waiting list mainly from Devizes Hospital would be resumed shortly.

1949 TO 1956 BOARD OF CONTROL INSPECTIONS

These inspections give a snap-shot picture of the conditions. The total number of beds in the hospital was 199. A tea party and canteen was held in the dining hall twice weekly, organised by local ladies. Patients were able to buy tea and cakes and other goodies and have a social party. The new canteen was of great interest to the patients and also pleasing to Alec Bailey who had been in charge of the kitchen from 1945 (He served in this capacity until he reached retirement age in 1978).

The link with the outside world was considered to be admirable with fortnightly cinema programmes and a weekly walk. An outing to the seaside had taken place in the summer. Pocket money of 6d to 2/- per week was given. A new recreation area for the male patients was being laid out and the Red Cross was starting a patient's library. There were Occupational Therapy sessions involving rug making and leatherwork and a chiropodist held twice weekly sessions. Staff for the ward housing mentally deficient inmates were 6 male and 2 female nurses during the day and 1 male nurse on duty at night. There were 24 male and 15 female mental defectives, some on licence from Pewsey Colony. Entire segregation from other inmates of the hospital was impossible but the defectives were kept as far away as possible and in the main had their own day rooms and dormitories. By 23 November the number of beds was down to 187, of which 20 were reserved for the Local Authority. There was little opportunity or necessity to segregate the certified patients – when they needed sick nursing they were admitted to the hospital ward otherwise they shared accommodation with the Local Authority residents. The day rooms are described as well warmed and of cosy appearance with modern fireplaces, easy chairs and attractive curtains.

A 1951 report mentions that the patients were occupied in the garden, laundry and in housework as well as undertaking small odd jobs with some of the men doing part-time work outside. A few of the patients who did useful work received 2/6d a week pocket money, others only got 6d but the women had their sweet ration and the men their tobacco. May 1952 just 1 female patient was detained under the Lunacy Act but there were also 24 male and 14 females listed as mentally deficient on the books with 2 female patients on licence – one as a maid to the matron and the other as staff dining room maid. It was suggested that the rate of pay/pocket money should be increased. There were 4 boys out in daily employment and they were allowed to keep some of the money they earned.

A certain number of the inmates were defined as being mentally deficient. These were people who would not benefit from being in a mental hospital and were not curable.

In 1953 inmates included 23 men and 14 women plus 40 certified mentally deficient. It was recorded that Dr Varian visited daily, there was a weekly dental surgery and an Occupational Therapist and Chiropodist were employed. By May of 1955 all the female certified patients had been removed and 7 males transferred elsewhere leaving just 16 male certified inmates, all over 16 years of age. The changes meant that the defectives had to live upstairs in three wards with only one day-room which they had to share with other types of patients.

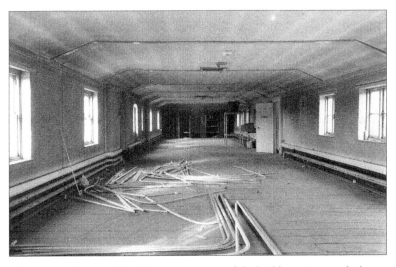

Dormitory for mentally defective boys at top of the building. Even in the late 1980s the walls were unplastered as can be seen from the brickwork

The inspector considered that the defectives being scattered around the building was unsatisfactory. By August 1956 the number of mentally deficient patients were down to 12 but the accommodation was still not thought to be satisfactory. In spite of this they were said to be comfortable and enjoying the amenities such as T.V. and the occasional coach party together with escorted cinema visits. Three of these men were out at work and they contributed 12/- per week from their earnings for their maintenance at the hospital. Apart from

Occupational Therapy most of the other inmates did work such as coal-portering and domestic work in kitchens and wards. Again it was pointed out that the monetary reward for this work was rather small. At this time considerable rebuilding and decorating was going on in the wards leading to disordered quarters.

Back to the Guardians' Minutes.

1952

'The hospital gives an impression of a homely informal place due, I am sure, to the personal interest in the patients as individuals taken by Mr Howell and Mrs Howell the matron'. Every three months the institution was visited and reported on by various local people.

1954

Mid-Wilts Management Committee appointments were made including the Craig-Howells for Management and George Waistell as representative for the domestic staff, 14 members in all, 7 of whom were to be members of staff.

The aims of the Committee were to give staff a say, to prevent friction and misunderstanding, deal with hours of work, holiday arrangements and to consider any rules affecting the staff.

Various problems came to light once members of staff were able to comment on conditions. Their initial reports say that the toilets in the sick ward block were inadequate (just 4 for 51 patients). It was pointed out that there was no money available but it would be kept in mind. Also there was no staff toilet on the sick wards. The reply was that there was a toilet nearby which could be used in break periods and if necessary staff were permitted to leave the ward, the toilet only being 50 yards away.

A member of staff commented that heating on the sick wards was inadequate for the patient's welfare. Temperatures had been checked and were 57-60 degrees on the ambulatory wards and 54 to 60 degrees on the sick wards during the previous January cold spell. It was agreed that the temperatures were not good enough but improvements would have to wait for money to be made available and staff were asked to ensure that heat was not lost through open doors and faulty windows. Many of the staff comments were not followed up, all for the same reason, no money was available.

The subject was brought up that each nurse had to serve 25 breakfasts between 7.30 and 8.00 a.m., which included feeding the helpless cases, clearing away and stacking dishes in the ward kitchen. The less than helpful comment made was that the staff needed to co-operate with the different shifts. Other suggestions were not seen as appropriate to be brought before the Committee as Matron should have been approached first. Work at the sick wards was very heavy largely due to a tendency of outside doctors to send their border-line cases for treatment.

1956

Staff shortages (trained personnel) were so severe in the latter half of December that all admissions had to be stopped.

1961

After Christmas immediate pressure occurred on the bed state. Devizes Hospital was severely blocked by geriatric patients but few St James patients were well enough to be transferred to an ambulant ward and only then if no stairs were involved. The same problem still existed for male patients even by April 1962.

1962

In this year the Regional Hospital Board announced that St James would be closed and replaced by a new geriatric Hospital.

No deaths or serious illnesses during the festive time. Redecoration completed very satisfactorily especially improvements in the downstairs toilet facilities for the male wards which used to be so dingy and depressing, but the M.O. pointed out the battered paint and woodwork elsewhere.

1963

The nursing staff were complimented on the wonderful morale existing amongst the patients, many of whom were only kept mobile by the constant exertion on the part of the nurses. This had led to a number of patients being recommended for hostel accommodation. However, the female waiting list was longer than ever with many elderly ladies waiting to be transferred from Devizes Hospital. The reason might be the unusually low death rate at St James and also the fact that hostel accommodation vacancies occurred very seldom.

1964

In July a patient caused an administrative problem. Certified by the Medical Officer as fit for Part 3 accommodation this one-legged man who lived a wheelchair existence refused to leave the hospital. The area allocated as a Part 3 Ward at St James was unsuitable for a wheelchair. Expulsion from the hospital was considered to be distasteful and could attract adverse publicity therefore it was decided that the matter be discussed in Committee.

(Under the terms of the National Assistance Act of 1948 it became the responsibility of Local Authorities to provide accommodation for adults if they were disabled or in need of care and support, this was known as Part 3 Accommodation. At this date Southfields in Victoria Road, Devizes was available for this purpose).

1965

Because of the increasingly heavy work-load an Assistant Matron had been appointed. This had helped but the difficulty now was a shortage of Ward Maids.

1966

By July new showers were in use proving a great success. Most patients liked them as it involved them in far less physical effort. The same for female wards was to be considered.

1967

A patient, suffering from a chronic depressive illness, climbed through the dormitory window when unobserved and fell to the courtyard below. She suffered a severe fracture dislocation of the left ankle and was to be transferred to Roundway Hospital when well enough.

1968

An extension of the internal telephone was needed on Ward 1. The constant demand of the telephone had increased staff work as they had to negotiate 2 flights of stairs.

In July work on installation of a lift had begun and would permit more movement of patients and more use of the hospital grounds in the summer.

1970

The Buildings Committee assessed the proposed scheme for a sun lounge – it was hoped that work would start soon. It was noted that Mr Kemp's enthusiasm for the project had been largely responsible for its existence. The M.O's report indicated that work started on the project at the end of the year.

1971

This year saw the start of discussions about a possible new building with improved rehabilitation facilities including both a bedded unit and a day hospital. Limited funds were available but there was a small amount of money in the Amenity Fund that could be used for urgent needs. The Regional Hospital Board was shortly to start planning for a replacement hospital, possibly to start in 1975/6. The Committee proposed that a temporary day hospital be established in association with the new physiotherapy department to assist with the run-down of patient numbers. The Physiotherapy department was provided at a cost of £1,000 in April 1972.

The sun lounges for Seymour and Philip wards were nearing completion and there was to be an official opening ceremony on 11 July when the lounges would be declared open by the wife of the Chairman of the Regional Hospital Board. The Devizes Lions enhanced the opening by presenting some colour T.V. sets for the use of the patients.

1972

There was a meeting of local health officials for the three counties caught in the tangle over the Bath Clinical Area future. During this meeting it was announced that St James would be replaced by a 112 bed hospital on a site adjoining the Maternity Hospital and Roundway Hospital and work would start in April 1973. However in 1974 the Ministry turned down the proposal to rebuild St James on a site in the grounds of Roundway Hospital because it was against the policy to allow accommodation for the elderly in the vicinity of the mentally ill. Dr Varian worried that the reduced bed statistics occasioned by the opening of the new St James scheduled for 1975 were 'a bit sombre'. Staff were assured that an increase in welfare beds and support in the home would suffice. 'Integration with the Community' as far as the Medical Officer was concerned was 'a phrase viewed with deep distrust'.

In April redecoration work had been agreed for the 72/73 financial year amounting to £5,000 but this would have to be modified owing to the revised programme for the new hospital. It was proposed that the work for a new hospital should start on the site in April 1973 and to be operational in April 1975 with 84 beds. The number of beds proposed was increased to 112 after some concern was voiced whether this number would be sufficient but then reduced back down to 84.

The 40 hour week had come into operation at the beginning of January meaning that additional staff would be required and the members of the Committee wondered if there would be any financial help.

A description of nurse's uniforms followed. The dresses were semi-princess style with belt and adjustable Peter Pan collar in light blue, the same for untrained staff but in yellow. A request for cloaks for the nurses was turned down as there were communal cloaks available on the wards for use by staff who had to escort patients. It was at this time that it was decided to have a staff magazine or newsletter and Sister Murray agreed to be the editor.

A staff dinner and dance was held in January – a very happy affair.

1973

In October there was no final decision from the Regional Hospital

Board, which had taken over the Bath Clinical Area, about the new hospital. During January a visit had been received from a member of the Hospital Advisory Service. The M.O thought that the reduced bed numbers proposed for the opening of the new St James Hospital scheduled for 1975 was worrying.

1978

Reported in 'Reflections' (the Devizes Hospital Magazine) by John Coles, Sector Administrator, that steps were in hand to improve St James and included plans to provide a day hospital.

1980

A meeting of all heads of departments was arranged to discuss the concept 'Could we do better in the future' as no one had anticipated how deeply questioned the original ideas and aims would be. Everyone thought that it was most important that patients retain their identity and dignity, particularly high dependence and terminal care patients. Down to earth John Coles thought it important that patients should have more privacy wherever possible for toilet and bathing facilities.

1986

In his foreword to the booklet *Changed Times* Dr David Wright, Consultant Geriatrician, said

> What of the future? The building is showing its age, both in design and structure so in the long term it will have to be rebuilt. In the meantime there are several developments that we would like to see such as a 'day hospital' where treatment can be given without the distress of admission to a hospital bed.

In 1988 it became necessary to close part of St James as it had failed to meet safety regulations. The implications of that decision were explained to the staff.

Sadly, within just a couple of years the site was derelict.

THE END OF THE HOSPITAL

1990

5 July. Councillor Gudrun Collis suggested a march around Devizes to protest against the closure of St James Hospital. Councillor Doyle thought that a protest should be taken to Bath to a meeting of the Authority to express the town's indignation. He accepted that there was a cash crisis and that 'in our wildest moments no-one can expect the Authority to change its mind about the St James Hospital closure on 30 September'. At a Town Council meeting on 6 September it was stated that Devizes was unlikely to get its promised new Community Hospital before 2000. Devizes M.P. Sir Charles Morrison promised to pressure Kenneth Clarke (Paymaster General at the time) to make money available to build a new hospital. At a public meeting at St Martin's Hospital in Bath on 12 September it was claimed that the closure would shorten old people's lives and Social Services gave a vote of no confidence in Bath Health Authority. A reliable medical source states that all of the patients who were transferred from St James Hospital at its closure died within the year.

The writing was on the wall well before this date – the number of staff had been reduced which meant that wards had to be closed and

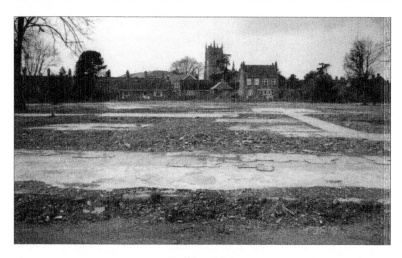

Bulldozed Site

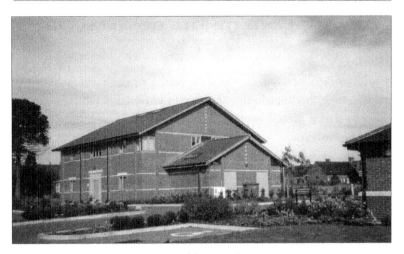

New Buildings on the site

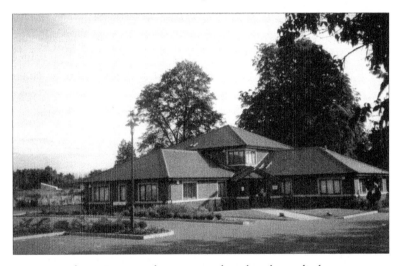

consequently patient numbers were reduced and very little money was made available for improvements and upkeep.

The staff naturally felt very upset about the closure and felt that they had had no say in the decision. Some obtained jobs in other hospitals in the area or became District Nurses whilst others did not go back into the nursing profession.

30 September – fait accompli – the 30 residents had already been transferred to Devizes Cottage Hospital and hospitals in Chippenham

despite the fact they were only supposed to be moved after the new hospital was built although it was impossible to say when that would be. As we know now that was never to happen. The Wiltshire Gazette listed plans for the derelict site after it had been bulldozed suggesting these could include three developments, almshouses, a charity headquarters and a doctor's surgery. This actually did happen.

12
Incidentals

The following are items which didn't fit comfortably into any other chapter.

1837

James Flower of Bromham, having been discharged the previous week, took away workhouse clothes, those he brought having been destroyed as useless. It was ordered that the cost of such clothing be charged to the parish of Bromham. Similarly, clothes taken by Eliza Grant were to be charged to Rowde.

In early February Ann Hampton who had been in the House for 12 months applied to be allowed out to visit her aunt. This was refused. The Board also refused to allow an inmate named Slade to go out to search for work. In May George Nash of St Mary's parish fared better. He was permitted to leave the House until midday to attend his father's funeral.

1839

8 October. Officers of the establishment were not to be allowed a different quality of tea from that generally used in the house.

1875

13 April. Constable Rich applied by letter for a reward for the apprehension of Cornelius Pike charged with leaving his wife and family chargeable to the Union. As it appeared Pike had not left the town and there was no difficulty in finding him the Board resolved it was not a case for a reward.

ESTIMATED WORKHOUSE EXPENDITURE FOR THE HALF YEAR ENDING MICHAELMAS

Maintenance	£40
Out-relief	£2,610
Lunatics	£650
Rations	£90
Medical	£120
House	£90 (Furnishing and repairs)
County rate	£625

1878

In June Mr Akerman had resigned his post as Assistant Overseer for Bromham and had requested refund of his Bond. The Clerk was directed not to give it up until after Mr Akerman's accounts had been received.

1882

11 July. The Board agreed to sign a petition to the House of Commons in favour of the Government Annuities and Insurance Bill to enable persons to make cheap and secure provisions for old age and the support of their families.

1908

In September Sidney Walker Maidment had returned to the Workhouse and expressed his desire to join the army and the Board made arrangements for him to do so. Because he was under-sized for the army he was turned down so he joined the navy.

27 October - Army pensioners in the Workhouse had their pensions paid quarterly. The Board decided to wait until arrangements for Old Age Pensions were in working order before deciding what they should pay towards their keep. Mr Haldane questioned why they were in the Workhouse anyway.

1912

In December a letter was received from the architect enclosing a certificate of completion of the new mortuary. Builder was W.E.Chivers.

1914

February. The supervising of inmates — copies of recommendations were to be posted up in the main wards. This was to show both staff and inmates what their rights and obligations were.

1927

A note in the Minutes in May show how closely expenses were monitored. There is an entry in the accounts noting a refund of 5d overpaid by the Union to one of the shopkeepers.

A tender to supply various materials gives an idea of the inmates' clothing. Items purchased included striped shirting, grey serge, coloured print, fine calico, flannel and muslin.

A circular letter was received from St Thomas Union which contained a resolution expressing the opinion that Chairmen of Parish Councils should be authorised to grant temporary relief in cases of sudden or urgent need and inviting the Board to support this resolution. After discussion it was resolved that the Board was not willing to support this proposal and no action was taken.

1930

Tenders received for snuff and tobacco and laundry items. Clothing requirements show that socks and stockings and vests were required but there is no mention of other underwear!

1966

In October 50 tons of block limestone had been ordered and was at the Wharf awaiting collection. An advert had been placed in the Labour Exchange for 3 married men with children for stone-breaking at 2/- per ton. Some local citizens complained on behalf of the unemployed about the poor rate of pay.

PAYMENTS BY RELATIVES

1874

A letter was to be sent to say that if Amelia Perkins entered the Workhouse application should be made to her husband for repayment of cost of her relief. The Order was rescinded – she was entitled to relief.

22 December. Charles Bridewell of Potterne was ordered to pay 6/- a fortnight towards maintenance of his wife. (In the quarterly accounts there is a list of people paying between 1/- and 12/- for their relatives).

1916

In October a 25 year old man had been taken from the Workhouse to the National Hospital for Relief and Cure of the Paralytic and Epileptic in Queen Square, London, but had been sent back as incurable and therefore not fit for admission. An interested member of the family had contacted the Turner Memorial Home of Rest at Liverpool to see if they would take him. In the mean time John's father had written to the Board asking for a reduction in the maintenance charge. This was refused and the Collector was instructed to proceed to enforce the order obtained against him.

1923

25 September. A.Griffin returned clothing in which he went away and remitted a further contribution towards the maintenance of his wife and children.

1927

8 February. William Fisher and wife Edna had been transferred. The full amount of the man's pension was 18/1d per week and should be claimed towards cost of maintenance. Edna was practically destitute so further information was required before a decision was made on how much they would take.

NOTIFICATIONS OF MARRIAGE

From 11 October 1836 Guardians were given the right to register marriages for the Devizes District (St James, St Mary's and St John's). Other districts were given the same rights.

On 31 January 1837 a room was to be rented for one year for the purpose of a Registry Office subject to the approval of the Registrar General. The Clerk was directed to fit the same up in a proper manner and to purchase all necessary books, forms, boxes etc. at the expense of the Union.

Just a few intended marriages are listed in the Minute Books.

CHAPEL AND CHAPLAINS

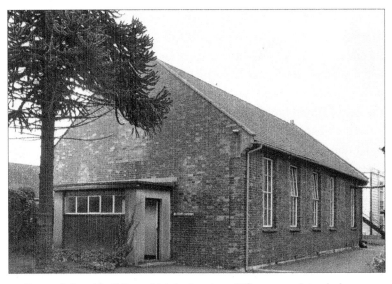

Original chapel building which had various different uses through the years

An 1860 publication *Union and Parish Officers Almanac and Guide* lists the duties of the Chaplain – to read prayers and preach a sermon to the paupers and other inmates of the Workhouse on every Sunday and on Good Friday and Christmas Day. He was to examine and catechise children belonging to the Church of England at least once a month and to keep a record of this and to look out for the moral and religious states of all the inmates. He was also required to visit the sick paupers and 'administer religious consolation'.

1874

14 April. A letter was received from the Protestant Alliance about Roman Catholic Chaplains which asked the Board to petition against a Prison Ministers Bill which enabled the Secretary of State to appoint Roman Catholic chaplains where ten Roman Catholic prisoners were under detention. The Board agreed to petition against this Bill possibly because they feared that the same proviso could be made for Workhouses and could cost money.

1915

26 January. The Chaplain reported that there was an insufficient number of prayer and hymn books for the inmates attending the services, also a new bible was required. Mr Young offered to provide the prayer and hymn books. Regarding the bible it was asked if the present one was beyond repair. The Reverend Kingsland was asked to find out but in the mean-time the cost of repair was agreed.

9 February. The Reverend Kingsland had made enquiries about the use of the 'Apocrypha' at Church services. Not obligatory so the Committee decided not to provide copies.

KINDNESSES

At the start of the Poor Law Amendment Act no extra food was to be allowed on Christmas Day and definitely no alcohol at any time unless prescribed by the Medical Officer but by 1840 extras were allowed as long as they did not have to be paid for by the Union. There were regular reports in the Minute books of various acts of philanthropy including concerts, teas, and entertainments for the residents and there were treats on Christmas Day from the start despite the regulations. The Poor Law Commissioners did authorise Christmas extras in 1847 although in 1884 there was still the proviso 'no alcohol'.

1838

19 June. Dinner of beef and plum pudding with one pint of good ale for adults and half a pint for children to be allowed in order to celebrate the Coronation.

1874

George Bullock of St James parish was allowed by way of loan the cost of a truss for his wife and the Collector was required to obtain repayment by reasonable instalments.

1882

21 February. An application was made by the mayor of Devizes on behalf of Miss Coward that she might be permitted to leave newspapers of a pictorial and non-controversial character at the workhouse for the amusement of the paupers. The board sanctioned the *Graphic, Illustrated News, Pictorial World, British Workman, Sunday at Home* and *Leisure Hours,* on provision they were left by a person who was disposed to supply them, it being clearly understood that there was no obligation to return them.

1905

In August inmates were taken on Roundway Hill to spend the day. Cakes were provided by Mr Drew, Mr Meek gave mineral water and Mr Smith a cask of ale. Others sent fruit and magazines and papers. At the end of November Mr Robbins asked permission on behalf of the Mayor for the able-bodied inmates and children to attend a pantomime at the Corn Exchange during Christmas week.

A further entry lists gifts given by benefactors. These included sweets, oranges, figs, nectarines, bon-bons, toys, flags, evergreens, Christmas stockings, cakes and tobacco plus 6d for each child.

1908

Grateful thanks were sent from the Committee to Mr and Mrs Berry for 'so hospitably entertaining the inmates to tea at Allington' and also to Miss Colston for providing tea and presents at their house. (The Colston family regularly gave the inmates tea parties at Roundway

House over the years). Also received had been many gifts from the Ladies Visiting Committee to the inmates.

1909

Christmas day. The Master was pleased to convey to the Board the inmates' thanks for a very happy day and for their Christmas dinner. This entry was followed by a list of gifts and donors.

1914

There had been excellent entertainment for the inmates, with a most successful concert by Madame Clara Butt on the 18 December (this was before she became a Dame). The Board was indebted for her thoughtful generosity. The Board Room had been arranged for the occasion and Mr Matthews had gratuitously fitted extra gas jets (he later sold these to the Board for £2.15.9d).

29 December. On Christmas day the inmates had spent a very happy time and wished to convey their thanks to the Board for providing them with their Christmas dinner. Gifts were received of oranges, sweets and grapes, chocolate, crackers and tobacco from the Mayor and Mayoress and other townsfolk who gave crackers, sweets, oranges, tobacco, a cask of ale, mince pies, evergreens and books.

1916

Sunday-School children and friends of the new Baptist Chapel gave a service of song which the inmates had enjoyed. The Guardians gave them hearty thanks.

In October Miss Colston had organised tea and amusements for the inmates on the green plot in front of the infirmary.
Messrs Stratton Sons & Mead gave a parcel of bananas and also some grapes from the St Marys Harvest Thanksgiving service.

In November it was decided that the usual Christmas fare be served taking into account the Masters discretion regarding economy. He was also to arrange suitable entertainments. Mr A.Matthews had offered to give his usual New Year show and this was welcomed by the Board.

1921

The Committee passed a hearty vote of thanks to the manager of the Picture Palace for a free entertainment given to the inmates of the house who were able to accept his kind invitation. The manager of the cinema continued to offer treats and by 1952 inmates could visit the cinema weekly (free admission) plus a cinema show was given once a month in the hospital with entertainments at least once a week. These were held in the men's dining hall but there were plans to convert the chapel into an entertainment hall, but by the St James Hospital days this had become the staff canteen.

1922

March. The Master was given discretionary power to serve out tobacco to the inmates according to, what in his judgement, they were entitled to receive.

1927

A letter was received from Devizes Liberal Club offering to arrange for the Club's Concert Party to visit. Offer accepted. A note followed saying that Miss Colston and her mother had arranged tea for the fiftieth time.

The Health Inspector in his report described two nice shelters in the garden where the men could sit and smoke. Visitors were allowed every day and the House, in his opinion, was run on very friendly and kindly lines.

1948

Efforts were being made to improve recreational facilities for the patients. To help with this a set of bowls was donated by the Devizes Bowling club.

WORK FOR INMATES AND CASUALS

The term 'Workhouse' was meant to alert the able-bodied that they would be expected to do work if admitted – hard and repetitious work and not for the work-shy.

1836

Colonel A'Court to be asked about suitable employment of able-bodied paupers. His reply in November made the suggestion that suitable tasks were picking okum, making paper bags by the women and making skewers by the boys. The Board decided to look into bone crushing and the Clerk was to find out what equipment would be required.

1837

Colonel A'Court wrote concerning an application to the Alderbury Union for the model of a bone crusher used there. At a September meeting the Board decided to order one of the machines 'without delay'. This was done on 4 September and it arrived in Devizes on the 9 Oct. The Master was directed to find out what price they could expect to get for the crushed bone. Nothing in the Minutes suggests that the crusher was ever used in Devizes.

The scandal at the Andover Workhouse in 1838 meant that national newspaper coverage brought the treatment of paupers to the attention of the Government and bone crushing was abolished. The book *The Scandal of the Andover Workhouse* by Ian Anstruther, describes the awful conditions and treatment that the paupers in the Andover Workhouse had to suffer.

1838

It does not appear that the Board had actually decided what work should be carried out as by the end of the year they were still considering the best way to employ paupers in the House. Various types of work were investigated. Oakum picking (old ropes cut into lengths and unravelled ready to mix with tar to caulk ships) and stone breaking were mainly used for casuals, the stone could be sold off for road making. Later entries in the Minutes show that stone breaking and cutting up old railway sleepers for firewood were tasks undertaken both by the fit and less able inmates and vagrants in Devizes.

Types of work felt to be suitable for women were mainly domestic and nursing duties.

Many Workhouses had land on which they could grow vegetables for use in the House and this was considered a suitable job for boys to undertake. The object of all the different types of work was mainly as a deterrent to admission but could also provide some income. This would be used towards Workhouse costs as no pauper was allowed to get compensation for his labour – his board and lodging in the Workhouse was his reward.

Although frowned on by the Central Authorities workers might be allowed extra tea, food and even beer, but this was not for casuals and vagrants, they had to do their tasks for bed and breakfast.

1842

The Master had power to allow men to go out looking for work but they had to get his permission first.

1918

The Master enquired about the wishes of the Board regarding giving a few of the old men who performed work of a disagreeable nature in connections with drains, cesspits etc., some reward. It was unanimously agreed that extra beer and tobacco should be allowed.

As late as 1927 it was noted that female inmates, except old ladies, were doing work of some kind such as sewing, laundry and scrubbing.

EMIGRATION

The 1834 Act allowed payments to assist emigration to be made from over-populated parishes. This was not necessarily abroad but could also be to the new industrial towns. This was up to the Board of Guardians to organise. On the 11 January 1836 the Minutes record correspondence with a Mr Moggeridge, emigration agent at Manchester. In April of the same year the Board ordered that a sum of money to cover expenses be allowed to the parish of Urchfont for the cost of emigration of some paupers, the sum of money required and the names of the paupers to be supplied. This was followed up in July when the Guardians of Urchfont parish applied for an order to send James Hale, Ann his wife and their nine children to Leeds.

The Clerk was directed to communicate with the emigration agent at Leeds. An earlier entry in June details the receipt of a letter of Isaac Romani who had been sent by the parish of Urchfont to Bradford in Yorkshire.

19 July. The Board consented to Daniel Ford, his wife and nine children to be sent to Leeds at the expense of Market Lavington parish. Another entry in March 1837 lists a request from Urchfont to send two paupers and their wives and children abroad as emigrants, the men are named as William Gilbert and Isaac Cook .

By May the Board had ordered 150 copies of a handbill, sent to them by Thomas Estcourt giving details of emigration to New South Wales, to be printed and circulated around the parishes in the Devizes Union. In early 1839 Mr Cook applied on behalf of George Amber, for assistance to emigrate. £5 was allowed, chargeable to St.James.

1914

The Guardians were reminded that money could be spent on any orphan or deserted child under 16 towards emigration costs and this was chargeable to the parish of settlement. The Dominions were felt to be of greatest benefit but costs for the USA were not allowed.

SUPPLIES

1875

Quotations received for supplying Guinness Stout varied from £1.5.0d to £1.7.0d for 10 gallon kilderkins and Wadworths gave a figure of £7.4.0d for 18 gallons of stout equal to Dublin.

1905

The tenders received on a regular basis give a good idea of the diet, clothing etc. In September of the above year they were requested for the following items:

> Flannel, Silesia (a twill weave fabric for pocket linings), unbleached linen and calico, muslin, winter serge, fustian (a heavy cotton material for men's clothing), flax and stout hessian. Hats (men and women's),

stockings (boys and girls), caps (men and boys), men's hose, cloth coats, cord trousers, boy's suits, handkerchiefs, striped shirting, blankets. (Again no mention of underwear or nightwear).

List of foodstuffs:-

Bacon, butter, currants and raisins, oatmeal, treacle, sago, cheese, cocoa, mustard, lump and moist sugar, pepper, vinegar, salt, lard, milk.

Other items include candles, starch, blacklead, scrubbing and long handled brushes, soda, blue, yellow soap, borax, straw and barley meal and of course not forgetting snuff and tobacco.

DIETARY

1834/5

The Unions were given 6 model dietaries to choose from and from this date inmates could request that their food ration be weighed in front of them.

1836

At the end of the year one of the Guardians, Mr Box, gave notice that he considered that the dietary should be looked at, altered and regulated. This was further discussed two weeks later but no decision was made for some months.

1837

In September the Visiting Committee had recommended that more bacon and cheese be used in the House and in December the Guardians decided that they needed the advice of the Medical Officer about an appropriate diet.

1838

Early in this year a new dietary was again discussed. It was suggested that several cases of cutaneous disease (some kind of skin disease possibly scurvy as this can be aggravated by a deficiency of vegetables) could have been caused by the diet. It was decided that the quantity of meat and particularly cheese were larger than necessary and potatoes and vegetables too little. Milk should be given instead of gruel on one or two days and there should be fresh meat instead of salt meat or bacon at least once a week. The opinion of the Committee was that the greater number of paupers came from the rural population and they were accustomed to subsist on bread and potatoes with occasionally a little bacon. Therefore if the diet in the workhouse were more similar to the ordinary state of living and contained less liquid food it would be more likely to keep the paupers in good health than the present dietary. Whilst there should be a sufficiency of good and wholesome food to keep the inmates of the workhouse in good health it should be wanting in some indulgence or luxury within the reach of the industrious and independent labourer so as to make residence in the workhouse irksome and disagreeable to able-bodied paupers (less eligibility again). The Guardians looked at the dietaries of twenty three other Unions and were surprised at the great differences, particularly in amount of vegetables. A new dietary was to be prepared and after taking medical advice this was to be transmitted to the Poor Law Commissioners for approval.

1839

No more than 8d a gallon to be paid for beer used in the Workhouse.

1846

A list of recommendations from London went out to all Workhouses and this listed bread, broth, milk or porridge for breakfast every day. Dinners should include items from the following list – bread, cheese, cooked meat, cooked bacon, soup, greens with suet or rice pudding. The paupers only got meat once or twice a week and bread and cheese were predominant over seven days a week, the pudding twice a week. Supper was yet more bread and cheese. Men got more bread, broth, bacon and pudding than women. The infirm could have tea for breakfast and supper with sugar and up to five ounces of butter a week. The Guardians were to direct what they felt to be an appropriate diet for under 9 year-olds and for children aged 9-16 - it was decided they would get the same as women.

1877

Tenders were accepted for preserved mutton and beef from McCall & Co and the Australian Meat Co.

1912

31 December. Because the stock of potatoes was nearly exhausted the Master was authorised to advertise for 8 tons of locally grown potatoes, that being the estimated quantity to last the season through.

1914

24 February. The Master was empowered to carry out the Medical Officers' recommendation and occasionally substitute jam or marmalade for butter. It was bread and jam or bread and butter, never both, but this was quite common amongst the working classes at this time. When the dietary was again reviewed in 1918 it was left to the Master to use his discretion in applying this rule.

Later in the year improved diets for both inmates and vagrants were to be put in place and they were to get meat or fish for five days a week.

1920

The Ministry of Health was no longer in charge of diet rates for regular inmates.

1926

In April there was an enquiry from Devizes Brotherhood asking why the price of meat for Officers was more than for inmates. The answer given was that the inmate's meat was English, of good quality and no complaints had been received. A tender dated March 1930 for supplying meat from Roses Butchers listed 'Inmates (English) 6d per pound. Officers (English) 1/2d per pound, so nothing had changed.

1930

A sub-committee reported in May describing how they had visited whilst inmates were having their mid-day meal which consisted of bread and cheese and tea. The only complaint was that some would have preferred beer with the meal.

Tenders were required for cheese, cocoa, salt, jam, Bovril, margarine, bacon, tea, rice, lard and moist sugar which gives some indication of the meals the inmates were offered somewhat changed from items listed in 1905 tenders for supplies.

13
Reminiscences

An extract from *Devizes Voices*, compiled by David Buxton entitled 'A Workhouse Boy'.

Elsie Watts. My grandmother was returning from shopping one day in 1933 when she passed a group of inmates from the Devizes Workhouse out on their exercise walk. They were brought out at a set time every day and they walked in crocodiles, one of boys and men and one of girls and women. When she got home she told me that she was sure that she had recognised one of her grandsons with them. We decided to wait until my father came home from work and then decide what to do. When he came home he said that if she was sure that it was him then we should go down there straight away and get him out. We went to the Workhouse and picked him out and after arrangements had been made he came to live with us. He was about 15 but as he didn't have a birth certificate and didn't know how old he was we had to choose a birthday for him. My grandfather said that we should pick 11 November 1918 as that was a day to celebrate, it being the date the war finished, so that became his birthday. I can't remember how long he had been living in the Workhouse but we found out how he had come to be there. He had been brought up in South Wales and my family had not seen him for a long time. When his mother died his father had chosen to keep his sister with him but had to admit Garry to the local Workhouse. The Workhouse people only gave support to people who were born in the parish so eventually he was sent to Devizes. He arrived in a hopeless state and didn't know us. He was not used to people being nice to him and it was a long time before he settled down. He was confused and cried a lot at first. He took a long time to get used to being offered food or drink when it wasn't a meal time. He joined the army when he was 18 but stayed with us until he got married. We became his family.

An Extract from *Hospital Diary*, by John Willett.

Nada & Douglas Craig Howell. St James was an old Workhouse and Public Assistance Institution which had unplastered brick walls when I arrived with my wife as Matron. We lived in the central tower block of the hospital. I had a long career working in Institutions and once handled 200 dossers a night and helped to bed down the Jarrow marchers in the 30s. The Devizes Hospital had a nursery for abandoned and illegitimate children, a wing for mental defectives and the rest for old people who had nowhere else to go. The plight of the babies was worst, they were all dressed alike in the most atrocious old-fashioned clothes, with outer garments of striped calico. Nada adds – I recall we bought proper baby clothes to the fright of the County Council because of the expense. We also insisted that the unmarried mothers took their babies with them when they went out, otherwise they might disappear and they were relied on as part of the work force. The hospital staff also took the children out for walks in huge prams and some of the children were terrified, they had never been outside the hospital before and screamed their heads off when they saw a horse.

Dr S.N. Varian. When remembering the early days at St James Hospital I recollect that I took over the medical care of the hospital when Dr George Waylen retired. The hospital was then in fairly poor shape, no money had been spent on it during the war years. The driveway which encircled the hospital was full of potholes which filled up with water on wet days. The biggest structural change was the building of the sun lounge. This was largely due to the great work of Mr Kemp the Chairman of the Management Committee in raising money for the building project

In the immediate post-war years there was a crèche for waif babies – I think we had about 20. They were housed across the inner courtyard. This part of the building was later converted into a day-

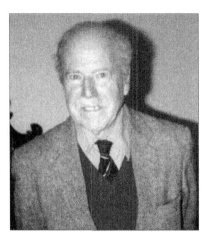

Dr. S. N. Varian. Medical Officer for St. James

room for nursing staff. In the male wing at that time they had a group of high-grade mental defective patients, several of whom were regularly employed in the town. They were later transferred to the Bristol area.

Over the years the improvement in nursing facilities and largely increased space for exercise led to greater activity by patients and a far higher discharge rate. This did not always meet with everyone's approval. I remember receiving a blistering letter from a doctor who found one of his most troublesome patients discharged home to his care!

Bill Underwood. After completing my National Service my first regular full-time job was at St James Hospital as barber. I shaved the men, some daily, some twice a week, cut their hair and also cut ladies hair. There was a small room near the porter's lodge which was designated as the barber's shop and ambulant patients came there. This was kept locked as I used cut- throat razors there but I used a safety razor on the bedridden patients. Talking about this brings back memories of the legendary Bertie Bushnell who visited the hospital weekly for a shave, usually done for free but occasionally he would pay a penny. I always found him rather disconcerting as he would gaze unblinking into my eyes as I worked. On one occasion he offered to collect used razor blades for me off the tip for a small fee!

Without knowing it any new staff underwent an initiation ceremony. They were taken round the various parts of the hospital in a formal manner ending at the mortuary (euphemistically called 'Rose Cottage' by the staff). There the body of an apparently deceased patient of the hospital would be lying upon a bier. On their entrance the 'body' would slowly rise up with a groan and say 'I aint arf 'ungry you'. The patient volunteer loved his play-acting role.

Many of the patients liked to tell me stories whilst I was cutting their hair. There was one particular gentleman called Harry Topp who had had been in the Wiltshire Regiment and fought in the Sikh wars. Strangely his mate called Steve Bowsher had served with him in the army and was a patient at St James at the same time. They were very close and actually died within a few days of each other. Another patient, a very well-spoken man claimed he had been batman to Maurice Chevalier.

Barbara Fuller. I worked for a short time at St James in 1966 as an Occupational Therapist. I presume they had no other applicants for the post as I was unqualified other than having worked as a clerk in the Occupational Therapy Department at Roundway Hospital. The O.T. room was very utilitarian and unattractive. The patients were happy to make patchwork cushions and curtains to brighten things up a bit before getting stuck into cane work and rug making. The cane work did prove a bit of a problem at first as when the cupboard storing the cane was opened quite a few cockroaches left in a hurry so it all had to be replaced.

There are two patients I particularly remember. The first was a nice old lady who would make us cups of tea and I believe helped in the kitchen. She had actually been born in the Workhouse and had lived there all her life. The second is an elderly gentleman who had had a stroke and I used to visit him on his ward to supply any necessary equipment for rug making, and watch while he did some work to make sure he knew what to do. This work had been prescribed by the doctor for therapeutic reasons. The next day I would be amazed at the progress he had made and the quality of his work – then I found out that during the night someone else, either the night nurse or another patient, would take over and 'help'.

Before the building was demolished a visit to look around, although it was interesting, was also rather distressing, the end of an era. Also one could get an idea of some of the conditions 'enjoyed' by the paupers. I particularly remember a large empty room on the top floor which had been the dormitory for M.D. boys. It had no plaster on the walls, just bare brick, there was a steep stone staircase with iron hand rails and what appeared to be very few toilet and washing facilities.

SOME ENTRIES FROM *CHANGED TIMES*

George Waistell 1940-1976 Male Mental Attendant then Head Male Attendant. There were no formal education requirements but a good testimonial from your previous employer was essential. My starting wage was £2.7.6d (living out). I had previously worked at Semington Institution and earned £45 a year living in plus 12/6d a week allowance for keep. The original sun lounge was built in 1971 by Vear's, largely through the efforts of Mrs Proudman and Mr Kemp. The great change came in 1948 at the start of the National Health Service. The Master and Matron, Mr & Mrs Balsh-Ward, were very kind to patients and very well thought of but they couldn't get the money to do the improvements they would have liked.

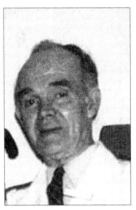

George Waistell. Male Mental Attendant 1940-1976

The large bell on the lawn was previously fixed to one of the walls. This was rung to warn that the doctor was coming and for the staff to get ready any patients that needed medical attention. The lanes at the side of the building were used as a 'bank' by the casuals as they had anything of value taken from them if they were admitted. In 1948 the sub-normal boys were given grey tweed suits with boots, striped shirts and nightshirts. They were better dressed than the staff. Prior to this date they had to wear institutional clothing.

The lino was polished with Ronuk. It was very slippery and today would have been considered a fire hazard. One patient who used Ronuk to get the fire going managed to set the chimney on fire. After the Fire Brigade had left he was very keen to get the fire going again! I wore a white jacket with trousers and an apron, sometimes a long white coat rather like a dentist. When I became a senior nurse I was provided with grey trousers. In my time the building was only locked up at night and, of course, the outside gates were also locked after dark. Children who were orphaned or neglected were looked after at St James's Home, the mentally deficient were dispersed to colonies such as Pewsey. Although the casual wards were closed there was always the odd chap who would come and ask if he could be admitted. As far as I know they were never turned away. These vagrants would be bathed but even so they were kept apart from the other inmates as they were often lousy. They would be given breakfast and sandwiches to take with them in return for which they would saw up old railway sleepers, make them into sticks and bundle them. At this time food was still weighed – everyone had their exact allowance but this was stopped soon after. Everything there now is changed times.

Mrs Peggy Dyke, nurse at 'The Home' 1932 – 1958. My first impression after interview and being accepted for 'The Home' in Commercial Road. I was taken to the sick wards – there were quite a number of people walking around in long print dresses of navy with a white stripe, all doing their various jobs. For example – taking around cups of tea to those unable to care for themselves. Slippers were allowed for these mobile people. From there I went to the 'Day Rooms'. There were two of these – one for the male inmates the other for female. They were equipped with wooden chairs but no cushions, they didn't come until later. The old were allowed to sit as long as they liked, the able-bodied had to work – very hard work, laundry, cleaning of the wards, waiting on the sick and infirm patients. Tea was served in large enamel mugs – badly chipped most of them. What impressed me most were the stone staircases, hard and most uninviting. The patients had to climb these stairs to get to their bathrooms – they were often very puffed when they got there. At the front of the building there was a large ward which housed the tramps. The nurses had a huge key, must have been about 18 inches long, to open the ward which was always kept locked at night. Working here was a little frightening to a young nurse at night but one grew accustomed to the nightly visits for the renewal of fomentations, taking of temperatures, according to the need of these poor souls who had to do odd jobs the next morning in payment for their lodging and breakfast. When the tramps came in they were stripped of their belongings until the following day or so until the able-bodied had performed their tasks and gone on their weary way. The tramps were of all types, some were well educated but had fallen on bad times. We worked as a team. Bright spots occurred from time to time. Tradesmen would give their time and transport to take those who were able to different beauty spots for an afternoon out – this was talked of for days. The late Mr Strong, also his son, brought unsold cakes and buns, chiefly at weekends. I think the Committee gave the names of St James's at the wish of the Matron, Mrs Balsh-Ward. She gave many years of service there together with her husband who was the Master. The staff were all very happy about the change of name. It was quite an uplift for the patients and visitors and we had a drink to this and felt grand. Worthy ladies of the town would visit and bring small gifts for the patients. The elderly stayed there until they died. If there was a relative willing to look after them they could go out but I never remember this happening whilst I worked there. The children were mainly illegitimate or had lost a parent. The tramps usually stayed for one night only – I don't remember any regularly coming back. Working hours – when on night duty you worked for three months with one day off. Wages in 1932 were just under £36 per annum all found. If you were on days you had one half day a month off duty.

Further memories were added by Mrs Dyke mainly referring to patients in the M.D. Wards. She says:

They were mostly women who worked in various departments of the hospital numbering about 20. The men, as I remember, were mostly elderly and walked around and around aimlessly but had the comfort of their little stock of tobacco. This was supplied to anyone capable of giving service such as looking after each other.

Sister Violet Murray. It was never the Workhouse when I started at St James Hospital in 1954. Things were already much improved since the National Health Service took over in 1948 and there was more money available and I have personally seen so many improvements both for the patients and the staff. At first Sister Sawkins and I were the only

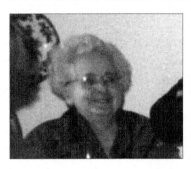

Vi Murray. Sister at St James from 1954

qualified Sisters – a little later on there were other part-time Sisters employed. I opened the male block which was previously occupied by the M.D. boys but there were still some of these boys on the top floor. The male sick dormitory was downstairs. There was only a tiny day-room – patients were either in bed or sat on chairs besides their beds. It was very crowded especially when visitors were here so the first sun lounge was a great improvement.

I remember that when I first started there were some very tricky steps down to the patients dining hall – no food lift then. Matron lived in a flat in the centre of the hospital, in my day Mrs Craig-Howell with Miss Clark as Assistant Matron. On Boxing Day Matron would ask staff on duty to her flat for tea. There was one patient I remember particularly – he had been on the Board of Guardians himself. He used to be in and out, would never stay for long but regularly turned up to be re-admitted. We would ring Dr Varian who was the hospital doctor and he would always say 'Take him back'. There was another man, a newly diagnosed diabetic, who had been told that whatever happened he must have his meals regularly. He was then sent home in an ambulance. Although he lived some miles away in one of the villages he was back in time for lunch and then he cycled home again. Another time I remember that Dr Renton came in and said that one of his patients had to get rid of a parrot – we had it for the men upstairs. It was a polite bird when it arrived but its language became a little rougher. We used to let it out of its cage but it became rather aggressive and used to try and peck the cleaner's legs so we had to find it another home.

The fetes were always well supported. Events for the patients were regularly organised, parties, bell-ringers and carol singers at Christmas. At Carnival time the Chippenham Crackpots always came around to entertain the bedridden. We had Harvest Festival, Red Cross Library, British Legion visiting ex-service patients – all sorts of things went on.

In the old days it was a threat – if you got into trouble you would go into the Workhouse. The present situation is based on good foundations from the time that it became a hospital. Some improvements emphasise this. Clothes for patients were obtained on approval from local shops. Any individual needs of the patient were passed on to Matron who would then inform the House Committee. Curtains replaced screens for the patient's privacy, alcoholic drinks given by visitors were approved by the doctor. The hospital was also a training school and therefore was regularly inspected by the General Nursing Council.

Mrs Jane King – nurse at St James's in the 1920s. Mr & Mrs Fear were Master and Matron. There were no pensions at that time and widows were often forced to enter. If a mother died leaving young children the father could leave them there during the week and take them home at week-ends. Dr Waylen was the doctor and called every day. Nurses earned £10 a year. Material for uniforms was supplied but they had to make their own. The uniform was a blue and white striped dress, ankle length, with a starched white apron and bib, a wide belt with keys hanging from it and a bonnet. Nurses had to buy their own cloaks. My brother-in-law was a member of the Board of Guardians – he was Mr Maslen the builder. People were separated by sex. On the female side there were wards for maternity (they had a good child survival record), a nursery for young children, old people and infirmary wards, but they also took female M.D's. The males had their own wards but there were no adult male M.Ds at that time. There were coal fires for heating protected by iron guards for safety. One patient named Charlotte used to pull back the guard and cook potatoes in the fire. Patients did all the cleaning and laundering – nurses only supervised. All food was cooked on the male side and brought over. Everyone's portion was weighed – a quarter pound of vegetables, half a pound of potatoes and a quarter pound of meat approximately. The nurses were not allowed to use their discretion in dishing up the food, it was strictly by weight but some patients did have special diets ordered by the doctor. I do remember steak and kidney pudding, boiled fish, salad was very rare. Pigs were kept by the hospital and ham could be had by the patients if the doctor arranged it with the Master. Tramps were put in rooms with no windows but with a sky-light. They had bunk beds. In the morning they were given a cottage loaf, a big piece of cheese and a hot drink of tea, coffee or cocoa. To pay for this the old had to work for one hour, the fit for two hours. On leaving they would produce 'tins' and were given a little dry tea and sugar and they would ask someone on the way to their next stop (usually another workhouse) for some boiling water. Discipline was very strict both for inmate and nurse. If someone sent a gift for one of the nurses it had to be handed in to the Master's office and entered in a book before they were allowed to receive it. Staff hours were long – six days a week with one evening off. We had to live in and be in by a certain time – if going to be late we had to get permission from the Master.

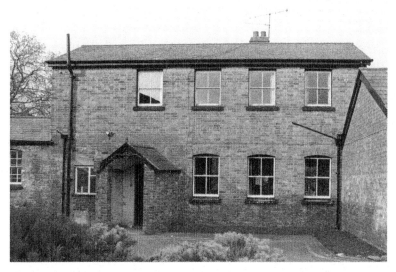

Children's Nursery, later nurses' sitting room and accommodation

The children had toys, I remember a rocking horse and slates and chalk. One patient was an excellent seamstress but was not very bright. She did the sewing and mending (beautiful darner) and received a small allowance and had the occasional extra such as a bar of chocolate. Another patient who had three illegitimate children was a good housekeeper. A man who needed a housekeeper wanted to employ her but they said she had to stay inside to pay for her children by her work. The man said he would take her on trial for one week and if she was alright he would marry her and also take her children. To keep everything proper she came back to the Workhouse every night. At the end of the week he professed himself satisfied and did marry her and was a good father to the children who afterwards did well for themselves.

I remember that Master and Matron lived upstairs. The nurses had an office and they also had bedrooms upstairs – they had to live in. Patients wore a one-coloured uniform of blue with aprons if they were workers. They had to do all the dirty jobs – the nurses never had to empty the bedpans. All possessions were taken away on entering. If they left quickly to work outside then they got their things back but otherwise everything was sold to help pay for their keep. Those who could work mostly did so inside. The wards had bare wooden floors which were scrubbed. Kitchen floors were also scrubbed and then covered with sawdust. We had our own church which the inmates used, they rarely went outside and then only with the Master's permission.

As a follow-on from Mrs King's reminiscences she herself became a patient in St James's Hospital in her and the hospitals latter years. In an article in the hospital newsletter (Reflections) she recounts how she had started work at the hospital at the age of 21 as a nurse when it was the Workhouse and very strict. After a long walk to reach work the hours were 12 per day with one hour off for meals and a comfort break. Staff had to clock in and money was stopped from wages if one minute late.

Duties included dealing with broken bones, burn blisters, faints, giving blanket baths.

After five years nursing she rebelled against having to have inoculations for various illnesses that were going round the villages covered by the Devizes Union. She got short shrift from the Guardians who said 'have them or be dismissed'. She decided to leave although the Guardians begged her to change her mind.

Miriam Smith. I was employed at St James Hospital from 1980 to 1990 as a Ward Sister. I was actually on duty on the day that the last few remaining patients were moved out to other hospitals. For some time there had been no new admissions and the hospital and its facilities had become quite run down. The patients, some quite ill and others for rehabilitation, were all housed in one ward but none of them wanted to go. However in the end they all went quite cheerfully except for one lady in particular who sat in a chair by the door and was adamant she would not go. The other patients had to sit in the ambulance until she eventually realised that she had no choice.

It had been such a lovely place to work and the staff were pretty down-hearted. Some retired early, other went to other hospitals or changed their occupations but none were made redundant.

14

Memories of Bertie Bushnell – Various Contributors

Bertie Bushnell, a man well known in Devizes in his time, regularly took advantage of the facilities of the Devizes Poor Law Institution and St James Hospital. Dr Varian described him as a character straight out of a Thomas Hardy novel.

In a report on his death in the *Wiltshire Gazette* the headline was 'his epitaph could be – Having no family he belonged to us in the community'. There were articles about him in the *Wiltshire Gazette* on 3 and 10 April 1980 following on from reader's letters on the 27 March, some affectionate, others not. The staff at St James hospital were in the first category and the records show that a japonica tree, dedicated to Bertie's memory, was planted in the grounds of the hospital. Whilst not listed as a vagrant in the admission and discharge register, over the years he was a frequent inmate of the Institution when he was unwell or the weather was particularly inclement. At his death in March 1980 the heading to the column in the *Wiltshire Gazette* was 'In memory of the legendary Bertie Bushnell'.

Described as a little man in an overlong overcoat and well-worn boots his full name was Herbert Nicholas Bushnell but he was known locally as Bertie. He was born on 8 May 1900 at Hare & Hounds Court, Devizes. His parents were Agnes Maud Bushnell née Burrows and Thomas Bushnell, general labourer.

Bertie could be a frightening man when he waved his stick around and shouted but that was usually because the children were taunting him. The above actions seemed to be the total of his aggression although his language could be rather ripe. However the above actions

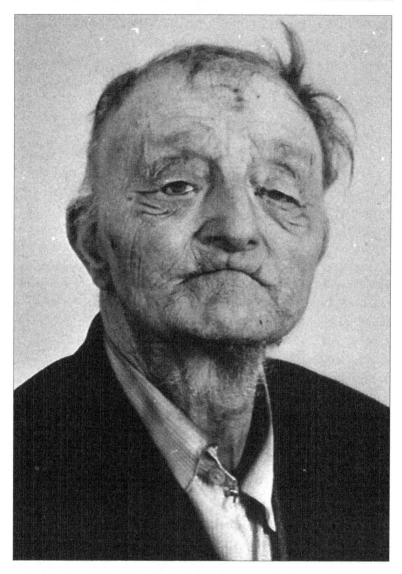

Bertie Bushnell – a regular visitor

were enough to make some of the children a little nervous of him but that did not stop some of the boys from teasing him.

There are numerous entries in the admission and discharge book for the Devizes Poor Law Institution. The first entry was when he was 27, admitted on 25 Oct 1926 discharged 15 Feb 1927. He was described as a labourer of St Johns. Others followed – aged 29, admitted 1 July 1927 discharged 8 September 1927; 11 November 1927 discharged 22 November 1927; 11 August 1929 discharged 10 September 1929; 24 March 1930 discharged 21 April 1930; 6 January 1931 discharged 31 Jan 1931. His periods of residence varied from eleven days to nearly four months and each time the records note that he was 'discharged at own request'.

He had other admissions to what became St James Hospital, turning up on a regular basis with the doctor for the hospital always saying, 'admit him'. He was just as informal in the way he left, purely to suit himself, to the extent that an overcoat and pair of boots were kept separately in Matron's office for him as he was quite capable of leaving in his slippers even if there was snow on the ground. The staff had to keep a close eye on him as he would smoke his pipe in bed and there were stories of close shaves when the bedclothes were also smoking! Tony Duck tells of his recollections of Bertie visiting his father's shop to buy 'twist'. This was used as either a pipe or chewing tobacco and was, of course, the cheapest variety.

Dr Varian told of a visit he had to make to Bertie when he was living on the tip at Stert. Bertie had dug a hole, lined it with whatever suitable material he could find and roofed it in with corrugated iron sheets. He was quite ill and Dr Varian had to get down on his hands and knees to crawl into the shelter which resembled a cave.

On 8 March 1941 Bertie married Emma Angel, widow of a local rag and bone man. He was 40 and she was 58. The certificate shows that he signed his name with an X but his wife was able to write her name. At the time he gave his occupation as labourer at the Gas Works and their address as Cypress Cottage, Gas House Lane, Devizes (now known as Lower Wharf, the cottage long gone). The marriage did not last and he even had an admission in 1942 for about 4 weeks which listed his wife as next of kin but rather sadly in 1949, when he admitted himself for approximately 8 weeks, he is shown as having 'No relation or friend'. Rumour had it that he slept with his boots on but it is more likely that he couldn't live with a roof over his head. A lady called Anna Rich, an employee of Devizes Rural District Council at the time, told of her surprise on being asked to be a witness to the wedding, his smart appearance being quite unusual, including the flower in his buttonhole. However, the ensemble was somewhat spoilt by the fact that he was wearing heavy boots (although they did appear to have been polished). Perhaps these were the same boots that he wore in bed! Emma had died in 1945 estranged from Bertie. She had tried to claim maintenance from him, even going to Court. She must have been an optimist and it is unlikely she ever got any joy!

Bertie died whilst a patient in Hospital on 8 March 1980. His death certificate gives his full name as Herbert Nicholas Bushnell, occupation as Farm Labourer (retired) and his address as St James Hospital, Devizes. He had pneumonia and heart problems. There was an attempt to get donations to give him a gravestone but this failed and today the site of his burial is just a grassy patch in Devizes Cemetery.

Terry Gaylard in his book *A Devizes Miscellany* adds some anecdotes describing Bertie as the super tramp and the last of the town's old cattle drovers. He described how he slept rough in makeshift shacks with other accommodation in an igloo-cum-wigwam, an old car body which led him to declare to a local lady that 'if I had wheels I wouldn't 'arf go'. Later he was provided with a caravanette by the Devizes Lions.

Because of findings during the research on Bertie an apparent mystery has emerged. It is not true that he had no relatives, he actually had a sister. She married and had children and after her first husband died moved to Market Lavington with her second husband and family. Her full name was Florence Georgiana and her birth entry gives the registration district as Pewsey. She was Bertie's only sibling, born in 1897. The census gives her place of birth as Milton in Wiltshire - probably this is Milton Lilbourne which would make sense with the registration district as the two parishes adjoin. In the 1901 census entry she was living in Devizes, 1, Hare & Hounds Court, with her parents and brother. Florence, also known as Florrie, first married in Devizes in 1919. Her husband died in 1930 aged 50 and she married again in 1932. Speaking to several members of the nursing profession and various Devizes residents it is strange that none of them knew or had even heard a rumour that Bertie had a sister! Despite much searching the last mention of Florrie is when she had a couple of short admissions in 1934 and 1935 by which time it was no longer called the Workhouse.

There are entries in the Devizes records of a Thomas Bushnell aged 65, occupation Hawker. He is noted to have a sister, Martha Bushnell of 174, Ram Alley, Burbage. In the 1901 census. Bertie's father is named as Thomas and gives his place of birth as Burbage. There was also an Agnes Bushnell who died 14 February 1922 aged 50, buried at Devizes and of St Johns Parish. Were these Bertie's parents, were they also inmates of the Public Assistance Institution? It looks possible.

Bertie was so famous or some might say infamous he even had a poem written about him

Bertie Bushnell, King of Drovers
Lying in a paupers grave
Left no wife or sons or daughters
Left no money, nothing saved.

Wandered thru' the lanes of Wiltshire
Driving cattle here and there
Sleeping by a smoking fire
Worldly things he did not care.

No tombstone marks his worn out body
Grass grows tall where he must lay
His body now returned to nature
His spirit roams the old byways.

Where'ere you walk near Etchilhampton,
Gypsy Patch or old Green Lane
Or if you walk down the Stert Valley
You'll tread the haunts of Bert again.

Bill Underwood

Bibliography

ANSTRUTHER Ian *The Scandal of the Andover Workhouse* 1973
BUXTON David – *Devizes Voices* 1996
CROWTHER M.A. – *The Workhouse System 1834-1929*
FULLER Barbara *Changed Times* 1986
GAYLARD Terry – *A Devizes Miscellany*
HIGGINBOTHAM Peter – *The Workhouse Encyclopaedia* 2012
LONGMATE Norman *The Workhouse* 1974
POOR LAW BOARD & HOME OFFICE – *Union & Parish Officers Almanac Guide* 1860.
WILLETT John *Hospital Diary.*
WILTSHIRE FAMILY HISTORY SOCIETY – *The Handy Book of Parish Law* 2004

Index of Names

A'COURT Colonel 12, 17, 19, 113, 175
ACKLAND Jane   98
ACUTT 146, 147
ADAMS George 135
    Mr 58
ADEY Mr 114
AKERMAN Mr 167
ALFORD Hannah 107
    Harriett 113
AMBER George 177
ANDREW Edwin 135
ANGEL Emma 196
ANSTRUTHER Ian 175
ARNOLD Edwin 94
ARTER Mr 115
ASHFIELD Thomas and William 125
ASHLEY Sarah 92
AWDRY Mrs Charles 36, 37, 47

BAILY Alec 155
    Mary Ann 75
BAKER Mr 18
BALSH-WARD Mrs 30, 66
BARREY Mr 114
BARTLETT William 125
BAYLEY Ann 122
BENNETT William 19, 115
BERRY Mr & Mrs 172
    V.J. 58
BIFFEN Emma 120
BIGGS Mr 58
BIRD Rev George 69
BLACKWELL Mrs 37
BLAGDEN James 104
    Mary Jane (also
        CROSSBRIGEMAN) 92
BLAKE Mr 125
BOND Rachel 67

BOWDEN Matilda 122
BOWSHER Charles 67
    Steve 185
BOX Mr 17
    Richard 110, 111, 112, 178
BRAIN Harriett 69
BRIDEWELL Charles 123, 169
BROWN Olive Margaret 28
BROWNING W 69
BULL Charlotte 95
    Elizabeth 75
BULLOCK George 103, 172
BUNDY William John (alias WALKER)
    97
BURDEN Mr 44
BURGE Mary Ann 67
BURGES Mr 33,
BURRY Betty 122
BURTON Freda 82
    Thomas 13
BUSHNELL Agnes Maude 193, 198
    Bertie 184, 193-8
    Florence Georgiana 197
    Martha 198
    Thomas 193, 198
BUTLER D.H. 58
    Daniel William 59
BUTT Clara 173
BUXTON David 181

CAMPBELL Rev. 36
CAPE A.G. 68
CARLESS W 115
CARTER John 143
CHAPMAN Stephen 28
CHILDREN (full surnames withheld)
    28, 29, 30, 35-47, 53, 88, 108,
    121, 181

CHIVERS Jemima 135
  W.E. 127, 168
CLARK Miss 189
CLARKE Kenneth 163
CLEVERLEY H.C. 71
CLOUGH John 68, 70
COLBOURNE Mr 95
COLEMAN Stephen 120, 121
COLES John 162
COLLINS William 135
COLLIS Gudrun 163
COLSTON Miss 172, 173, 174
COOK George 135
  Isaac 177
  Mr & Mrs 102
  Mr 24, 177
COOKSEY Seth 123
COOPER Thomas 75
CORNILL Leonard 143
COTTLE Fanny (alias FLOOD) 92
COUZENS Catherine 130
COWARD Miss 172
COX Frank 143
  George 66
  Thomas 136
  Mr 58
COZENS Ann and William A 13, 61,
  62, 117, 118
CRABTREE Miss S.E. 32, 68
CRAIG HOWELL Nada & Douglas
  66, 157, 183, 189
CRAWFORD Mrs 28
CREES Sidney Lacy 147, 148
CRISALL Rev 44
CROSS Henry 125
  Mrs 115
CROSSBRIDGEMAN Mary Jane (also
  BLAGDEN) 92
CROUCH Robert Peter 28
CUMMINGS Amelia 105, 106
  Mrs 105

DARK Thomas 136
DAVIES Mary Ann 63, 66
  William H 63, 66
DAVIS Benjamin 80
  Mary Golledge 67, 69

DIXON Emily 109
DOWSE Ellen Jemima 92
  James 93
  William 83, 95
DOYLE Councillor 163
DREW Mr 107, 172
DRISCOLL Charles 143
DUCK Tony 196
DUNFORD John 120
DURNFORD Charlotte 69
  John 68
DYKE Emily 70
  Peggy 30, 187

EARLE Mr 23
EAVES Mr 58
EDGELL Miss 47
EDWARDS 135
  Miss 114
ELLIOTT Clara 69, 148
  Edward 67
EMERSON Mr & Mrs 94
ENGLAND Henry Humphrey 68
ESTCOURT T.H.S.B. 11, 112, 177

FEAR Matilda 65, 67, 149, 190
  James R.K. 67
  William 64, 67, 149
  William Trevor 65, 66, 85
FERN T.W. 58
FERRIS T.W. 47, 58
FEW Annie 67
  Rose 67, 68, 70, 80
FIELD William Samuel 94
FINCH Mr 17
FISHER Alfred 99
  Edna & William 98, 169
FLOOD Fanny (alias COTTLE) 92
FLOOKS Mr 58
FLOWER James 165
FORD Daniel 177
FOWLER Mr 114
FOX Ethel 42, 69
FRANCIS George 93
  Henrietta 92
FRENCH John 18
  William 135

FULLER Barbara 185

GABRIEL Mrs 95
GARDINER William 124
GARRETT John 68
GAUNTLETT Ebenezer 93
    W.105
GAYLARD Terry 197
GERRISH Charles 120
GIDDINGS Arthur 67
    Mary Ann 92
    Mary Jane 92, 125
    Thomas 115
    Mr 58
GILBERT Ellen 91
    William 177
GILES John 67
    Mr 58, 128
GLASS John 12
    R.C.104, 105
    W 83
    Mr 105, 146
GODDARD George 109
    James 146
GORING John 14
GRANT Eliza 165
    Henry 125
GRAY Abraham 12
    George 81
    Mrs (GUY) 68
GRIFFIN Mr A 169
GULLIVER Jacob 123
GUY(GRAY) Mrs 68

HALDANE Mr 167
HALE Ann 176
    James 91, 176
HALLIGHAM William 135
HAMBLEN W.45
HAMPTON Ann 165
    Edward 75
    Emily 70
HARDING John 114
    Ralph 28
    William 18
HARTNELL Sidney 147
HASSALL Henry Jackson 34, 64

Jacob William 63
    Mary Tibbetts 34, 63, 64, 67
    Thomas 63, 67
HAYWARD Richard 120
HAZELL Henry 68, 117
HEAD Thomas James 17, 18
HEDGES George 136
HENLY Winifred 66, 70, 71
HENNIKER Lord 91
HERRING Harriett 67, 68, 69
HIDDER William 136
HILL Rev 58
    Richard 114
HITCHCOCK Dr Charles 74
HOBBS Emily Jane 92
HOLLOWAY Joseph 20
HOMES. Bath 44
    Bodmin 41
    Calne 27
    Croydon 38
    Devizes 114
    Farnham Royal 39
    Hastings & St Leonards 40
    Liverpool 169
    Newport
    Isle of Wight 29
    Purton 54
    Salisbury 37, 45, 53
    Sampford Peverell 41
    Stoke Park 35, 40
    Swindon & Highworth 54
HOOD Elizabeth 92
HOSPITALS. Arlesbury Asylum 94
    Hanwell Lunatic Asylum 92
    National Hospital for Relief of
        Paralytic & Epileptics 169, 114
    Roundway Hospital (Wilts Lunatic
        Asylum)84, 98
    St Barts 91
    Salisbury 109
HOWELL James 70
    Robert 70
    Sarah 82
HOY William 94
HUGHES Mrs 96
    Nora 84
HUSSEY-FREKE Mr 58

HUTCHINS Charles 27
  George 123
  Harry 124
  Robert 27
  Sarah 124
HUTTON Mr 95

JAMES Rev H.A. 69
JEANS Thomas Mark 64
  William 64
JEFFERIES Henry 143
JENKINS Mary 97
JONES Mr 27

KEEL Mary 109
KEENE Ernest 67
KELWAY James Robert 68
KEMP Mr 183, 186
KETTLEY Henry 70
KING Mrs Jane 190
  William 136
KINGSLAND Rev.J 145, 171
KOLLE David 75
KYRME Rev F.E. 69

LAVINGTON Robert 15
LEWIS David 19
LEWSINGTON Mrs 95
LONG Alice 68
  William 27
LOOKER Herbert G 68, 71
LOVELL Daphne 66
LOVELOCK W.J 148
LUCAS Ann 69
LUSH Fredk.M 39, 40, 58, 105

MAIDMENT Sidney Walker 167.
MARSH Nora 66
MARSHMENT Hannah 67
MARTYN Clara 67
MASLEN A 62
  William117
  Mr.58, 118, 190
MASTERS Isabella 84, 120
  William 68
MATTHEWS A 173
MAUDE Alfred 98

MAYO Emily 70
MEAD Samuel 81
MEEK W 58, 78, 93, 106, 172
MEREWETHER H.A. 32
MERRITT Henry 67
MILES Reuben 104
MITCHELL Mr 95, 147
MOGGERIDGE Mr 176
MOORE Mary 104
MORRISON Sir Charles 163
MORTIMER John 143
MURRAY Violet 188

NASH Elizabeth 122
  George 165
NEALE Frederick John de Coverly 69
NEATE Alfred E 68
  Ernest 81
NEEDHAM Sir Frederick 87
NEVILLE James 136
NORTH Kennerick 67
  Mary Ann 67

OATLEY John 79
O'BRIAN John 136
ORCHARD Robert 146
ORPHANAGES/HOMES.
  Birmingham 38
  Bodmin 41
  Bristol 40
  Calne 17
  Croydon 38
  Isle of Wight 29
  Liverpool 169
  Salisbury 37, 45, 53
  Sampford Peverell 41
  Stapleton

PARFITT Mary 67, 68, 69
PEARCE Dr.108
PEARCE Elam Jacob 67
PERKINS Amelia 169
  Mrs 115
PERRETT Susan 122
PETHRIDGE Amy 67
PETRAS Thomas 67
PHILLIPS Thomas 91, 114

PHILLIPS & WILLETTS Lunatic
    Asylum 114
PICKETT Robert 123
PIKE Betty 28
    Cornelius 165
PINCHIN Adelaide 27
PITMAN Mrs 95
POCOCK Joseph 67
PORTER Charles 118
POTTENGER Mr 58
POWNEY John 67
PRACEY Ms.94
PROUDMAN Mrs 186
PURNELL Benjamin 68, 70, 119
PURNIER Rev H 69

QUICK William George 68

RABY Dr 41, 42, 43, 46, 69
RAMPTON Maud 135
RANSOM Julia 67
RAYMENT Dr 96
READ William 32, 68
RENTON Dr 189
RICH Anna 196
    Constable 165
RIVINGTON Charles S 69
ROBBINS David 146, 148
    Elizabeth 107
    Ethel 122
    Mr.58, 172
ROBINSON William 135
ROGERS Frederick 143
ROLFE David 148
ROMANI Isaac 177
ROSE William 135
ROSE'S Butchers 180
ROUNDWAY Lord 148
RUSKIN William 136
RUSS Caroline 113

SAINSBURY Lucy 67
    Mr.58
SALMON, TUGWELL & MEEK 111
SANDERSON Jan 66
SARGENT Mr 58
SAWKINS Sister 188

SCHOOLER William 14
SIMMONS William 99
SLADE Jane 67
    John 20
    William 70
    Mr 58
SLOPER Edwin 12, 57
SMART Abraham 75
George 84
SMITH   Rev.A 114
George 135
    Heatherbell 68, 70
    John 66, 123, 137
    Julia E 67, 69
    Miriam 193
    Violet 28
    Mr 58, 172
SNELGROVE Mr 58
SPACKMAN Mr 15
SPRINGFORD William Henry 119
STARKY Mr 80
STEVENS Stephen 67, 68
STILES Samuel 66, 68, 117
STOKES Ann 123
STONALL Edith 81
STONE John 135
    William 68, 122
    Dr.109
STOUR William 67, 68, 70
STRATTON W 58
STRATTON SONS & MEAD 108,
    173
STRONG John 13, 68
SUMMER Mr 78

TALBOT Daniel 135
TANNER Jane 92
TAYLOR James 12, 80
TILLEY James 124
TONGUE Frederick 143
TOPP Harry 185
TRAVERS Rev 58
TRUMAN William 27
    Mr 15
TRUMPER Alice 71
TUCKER William 112
TUGWELL William Edmund 11, 18,

57, 111
TYLER Thomas 134

UNDERWOOD Bill 184, 198
   Elizabeth 67
   Maria 119
UNIONS.Alderbury 175
   Andover 175
   Bath 43
   Birmingham 109
   Bradford on Avon 108
   Bradford,   Yorks 15, 91, 177
   Brentford 93
   Bristol 86
   Calne 92, 108, 109
   Cardiff 97, 98, 99
   Chippenham 138
Clutton 92
   Cricklade & Wootton Bassett 96
   Gloucester 108
   Highworth & Swindon 50, 54, 108
   Islington 92
   Kensington 92, 109
   Lambeth 92, 98
   Lewisham 99
   Malmesbury 108
   Marlborough 123
   Melksham 108
   Merthyr Tydfil 98, 109
   Pewsey 97
   Plymouth 91
   Purton 96
   Reading 97
   St Albans 94
   St Marylebone 95
   Salisbury 108, 109
   Semington 186
   Shoreditch 92
   Southampton 93
   South Stoneham 97
   Southwark 98
   Trowbridge 108, 137
   Wandsworth 97, 99
   Warminster 139, 140
   Westbury 108

Willesden 98

VARIAN S.N. 69, 71, 89, 116, 151,
   152, 183, 189, 196
VEAR'S 186

WADWORTH's 177
WAIGHT Mr 95
WAISTELL George 157, 186
WALDRON Lovegrove 18
   Thomas 18
WALKER John (alias BUNDY) 97
WALTON-EVANS Miss 42
WARREN Thomas 143
WATTS Elsie 181
   Emily 67
   P.J. 59
   Sarah 66
WAYLEN George 69
George Swithen 18, 69, 71, 79, 121,
   183, 190
WEBB John 58
WEEKES Rev W.H. 69
WELLS Amelia 67
WENTWORTH Edward 93
WESTON James123
   Sarah 91, 107
WESTWOOD Richard 143
WHEELER Nellie G 67, 70
WHITE Benoni 14, 18
WILKINSON Mr 14, 17
WILLETT John 152, 183
   Mr 114
WILSON Sanders 63, 66, 113
WILTSHIRE Martha 63, 69
WITHERS John 12
WRIGHT Dr David 162

YARNOLD Daisy May 109
YATES Jean 66
YOUNG George 136
   John 18, 58
   Joseph 95
   William 58, 95
   Mr.171

Lightning Source UK Ltd.
Milton Keynes UK
UKOW05f1838061116

286984UK00009B/82/P